TLC for Parents of Seriously Ill Children

La Verne,

Oct. 26, 2009

Chad

May God bless you
and your family. Please
don't hesitate to contact
me anytime you need a
listening ear.

Rita Gray

Purposefully His,
Rita Gray
Psalm 46:10

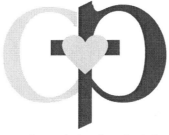

CarePoint Ministries ❖ Atlanta
www.ChristianCarePoint.org

CarePoint Ministries, Inc.
A non-profit faith-based ministry
www.CarePointMinistry.org
Atlanta, GA USA

CarePoint titles are available at discounts in bulk quantities. For details, contact the publisher at the above address.

Printed and Manufactured in the United States of America

Important Note: If at any time you feel you need to speak with a pastoral or professional Christian counselor, please call the church office for a referral to a member of our pastoral staff or a licensed professional Christian counselor. Church telephone number:

_____

Dedication

To parents past, present and future
caring for a seriously ill child.

Acknowledgements

I am so thankful to God:

for my family—Steve, my husband and best friend on earth; Katie, a beautiful young lady both inside and out; Ryan, a "Little Man" with wisdom beyond his years; and Chad, a child with a God-given strong will who taught me that surviving and thriving are possible while living with cancer.

for our Christian parents who taught Steve and me to trust in the Lord with all our heart and lean not on our own understanding; in all our ways acknowledge him, and he will make our paths straight (Proverbs 3:5-6).

for Mountain Christian Church Writers' Group. Trey, the servant leader who was obedient in beginning the group; Virginia, who held me accountable to a writing submission schedule and served as my mentor; Dawn, who prayed me through the project; Sally, who is the best public relations person anyone could ever have; and Glenn, who asked me the tough questions and expected answers.

for the moms of seriously ill children (Brenda, Christine, Connie, Kathy, Nancy, and Virginia) who I have laughed and cried with. I love you madly.

for the Kingdom Assignment at Mountain Christian Church and Virginia who shared her "talent" with me. I finally got it right.

for prayer warriors interceding on Chad's behalf while on treatment and on my behalf while writing this book.

for him allowing me to teach what he has shown me and to portray Jesus as the tender, loving Comforter to others who are on a similar journey.

for Kelly Hawkins' editorial skills and her gift of keeping all CarePoint writers unified.

for Scott and Lena Stewart's obedience to God's calling on their lives.

for his painful pruning in my life. May this book ooze with my love for you, Lord.

for the great things he has done! To God be the glory now and forever-more!

Contents

Introduction & Encouragement 11

Facts & Figures 15

Rita's Story 17

Week 1: Caring with TLC 23

Week 2: Caring for the Caregiver Emotionally 31

Week 3: Caring for the Caregiver Spiritually 39

Week 4: Caring for the Caregiver Physically 47

Week 5: Caring for the Clan Emotionally & Spiritually 53

Week 6: Caring for the Clan Physically 59

Week 7: Caring for the Seriously Ill Child Emotionally 67

Week 8: Caring for the Seriously Ill Child Spiritually 77

Week 9: Caring for the Seriously Ill Child Physically 85

Week 10: Caring for Our Future 93

Reading Section 103

   1 – Emotions 103

   2 – The Diagnosis 104

   3 – The Blame Game 107

   4 – Shattered Dreams 108

   5 – If 110

   6 – Fear of Death 111

   7 – Fear and Faith 112

   8 – Prayer 114

   9 – God's Promises in the Bible 115

  10 – Loneliness 116

  11 – Rest 118

  12 – Nutrition and Exercise 118

  13 – Real Friends / Support Groups 119

  14 – Attitude of Gratitude 121

  15 – Perseverance / Admit Our Weaknesses 123

  16 – The Diagnosis 124

  17 – Father / Mother 125

  18 – The Other Children 128

  19 – Home Sweet Home 130

  20 – Financial Needs 133

  21 – Insurance 134

  22 – The Diagnosis 138

  23 – The Prognosis 140

  24 – Attitude with a Capital A 142

  25 – Loneliness 143

  26 – Late-Effect Emotions 145

  27 – God has a Plan and a Purpose for Our Child 147

  28 – Sharing God with Your Child 149

  29 – Miracles, Faith, Hope, and Healing 150

  30 – Everything in Life Can't Be Fun 152

31 – Two Wonderful Things Our Children Deserve to Experience 154
32 – Life is a Party 158
33 – School and Your Child's Individualized Education Plan 158
34 – Play 161
35 – Survivor's Guilt 163
36 – Pain Management 164
37 – Thy Will Be Done 165
38 – Death—An Outsider's Observations 166
39 – Keeping the Memories Alive 168

Special Needs Ministry 171

References 173

Introduction & Encouragement

"'Come to me, all you who are weary and burdened, and I will give you rest.'"

—Jesus (Matthew 11:28)

First, let me say, "I am so sorry." My heart breaks for you. How I wish I could give you a big hug. I'm sure this workbook would not have been your number one choice of reading material. Certainly, it would not have been mine either. That is, before my son's accident and serious illness.

You have been on my mind almost ten years. Since my son's leukemia diagnosis, this workbook has been my heart's desire. This interactive resource allows parents of seriously ill children the freedom to address and work through the multitude of emotions we feel.

My prayer, as you work through the care sessions, is that at the very least you will not feel alone; but that you find hope in knowing that a fellow sojourner was sustained while traveling this rocky path. I pray that you receive encouragement and find a safe place to share your feelings with folks who are on a similar journey. At the very best, I pray you find the care and comfort you need through Jesus Christ, the tender loving Comforter of your soul, as you travel along this path of caring for your seriously ill child.

Each session includes a Bible verse that I urge you to commit to memory for the week. Ask God to weave the verse into the fabric of your life. Susan Miller of N.E.W. Ministries accurately says, "God's word brings hope, comfort and encouragement at any time, any where, under any circumstances, to any people, of any country! God's word breaks through lan-

My prayer, as you work through the care sessions, is that at the very least you will not feel alone; but that you find hope in knowing that a fellow sojourner was sustained while traveling this rocky path.

guage barriers, crosses cultures, unites hearts of different heritage, and heals international pain."

You will need a Bible. I quote the New International Version. Use whatever translation is easiest to understand.

Emergency situations arise when a Bible is not close at hand. Immediate comfort is available if we commit scripture to memory. God's Word offers a power that is not available anywhere else. Let's tap into God's prescription book to promote healing for our broken hearts.

The workbook is divided into ten weekly sessions. The sessions deal with three different roles we portray as parents.

Weeks one, two and three, are for us, the caregiver. Much needed and well-deserved tender, loving care is offered. Acknowledging and addressing the emotions that we initially feel as a parent of a seriously ill child is necessary. We must assess our feelings, our fears, and our faith.

These three caregiver sessions are first because we must attend to our emotions in order to effectively relate to our spouse, our other children, our ill child, our family members and friends, and the medical community.

In *Professionalizing Motherhood*, Jill Savage explains it this way:

> Have you ever been on an airplane and listened to the instructions about using the oxygen masks in an emergency? The flight attendants always give special instructions to those traveling with children: Put your oxygen mask in place before you place the mask on your child. Those directions seem to go against our very nature. Our first inclination is to take care of that child even if it means sacrificing ourselves. But when we stop to consider the reasoning behind the instruction, it makes sense. If we don't take care of ourselves first, we might not be able to help either one of us and we might both perish in those few precious moments. If we put our mask in place first, we are then in a position to care for others.
>
> The same principle applies at home. We must first take care of ourselves in order to properly take care of others. This will give us the stamina, patience, and perspective needed to care for the needs of others over the long haul (Savage).

Immediate comfort is available if we commit scripture to memory.

This reasoning is exponentially truer of a parent of a seriously ill child. First and foremost, address our emotions. Too often, the nature of this beast, a serious childhood illness, does not afford parents the luxury to do this needed exercise. I encourage you to take care of yourself.

Weeks four and five focus on caring for the clan. These weeks focus on the roles we played before and continue to play following our child's illness. Immediately following diagnosis, it seems as if life is standing still. The reality that life goes on can hit hard. These two sessions address dealing with those we love the most, our family. They, too, are hurting emotionally. This is a time when teamwork takes on a totally different meaning. All of our previous roles we played in life are still there and now we have even more new roles.

Weeks six, seven, eight, and nine deal with the caregiver role of the child with a serious illness. We focus on old and new roles and the new issues we may face with our children. Finally, week ten focuses back on us and our future.

Each week has devotions that are applicable to the lesson. In the next week's lesson you will find questions from the previous week's devotions. I encourage you to read the daily devotion and answer the questions in the next lesson. You will have the opportunity to share your answers during the next session. As a parent of a seriously ill child, we are bombarded with the physical aspects of the illness—the treatment, the doctors, and a whole new world in which we now reside. Please take the time to respond to the questions. Remember, don't side-step the other aspects of the illness. Deal with the emotional and spiritual sides, too.

Following each devotional, I encourage you to write a prayer in a prayer journal. Be sure to include a scripture in each prayer. Praying God's word back to him declares our confidence in his faithfulness in our lives. A prayer journal is an instrument of faith that allows us to periodically review how God's hand is working for his good in our life and our family's life.

Finally, I encourage you to choose a journal that you can use to record steps along your journey. Record the blessings along the way, too. Journaling is also a wonderful testimony of God's faithfulness in your life. As Joshua 4:7 instructed that the stones would serve as a memorial to the children of Israel of God's faithfulness to his people, so too, your journal pages will serve as a memorial of God's faithfulness to you, your family and your seriously ill child.

> Remember, don't side-step the other aspects of the illness. Deal with the emotional and spiritual sides, too.

May you rest in God's tender, loving care and comfort. Please share your journey with me. I look forward to hearing of God's faithfulness in your life as well as the privilege of praying for you and your family. My e-mail address is RitaGray@comcast.net. Please visit the TLC For Parents website designed for you at www.tlcforparents.com.

God bless you and comfort you on your journey,

Rita

Facts & Figures

Parents of Children with Serious Illnesses

We have one thing in common. We are parents caring for a child with a serious illness. Whether birth defect, life-threatening illness, or a life-altering accident brought us to this point, the result is the same. We are parents caring for a seriously ill child.

The truth is we are not alone. The enemy wants you to believe you are the only person dealing with this situation. Sadly, many parents are dealing with similar situations.

According to Candlelighters Childhood Cancer Foundation (www.candlelighters.org), "Each year in the United States, approximately 12,600 children under the age of twenty are diagnosed with cancer." The March of Dimes (www.marchofdimes.org) reports, "About 150,000 babies are born each year with birth defects. The parents of one out of every 28 babies receive the frightening news that their baby has a birth defect. Several thousand different birth defects have been identified."

Thankfully, more children are surviving life-threatening illnesses than ever before. Research and pre-natal care have boosted the chances of surviving a birth defect. Advancements in emergency medical care are increasing the numbers of people who survive accidents.

Therefore, palliative care is a term whose time has come in the medical field. According to the World Health Organization:

> "Palliative care for children represents a special, albeit closely related field to adult palliative care. Palliative care for children is the active total care of the child's body, mind and spirit, and also involves giving support to the family. It begins

The truth is we are not alone.

when illness is diagnosed, and continues regardless of whether or not a child receives treatment directed at the disease. Effective palliative care requires a broad multidisciplinary approach that includes the family and makes use of available community resources; it can be successfully implemented even if resources are limited. It can be provided in tertiary care facilities, in community health centers and even in children's homes.

"Palliative care improves the quality of life of patients and families who face life-threatening illness, by providing pain and symptom relief, spiritual and psychosocial support from diagnosis to the end of life and bereavement" (www.who.int/entity/cancer/palliative/en).

To that end, consider this workbook part of the palliative care for you and your family.

Rita's Story

You Wouldn't Believe Me If I Told You

"Do you want to talk in front of Chad or go to a different room?" the doctor asked. Chad, sensing something was wrong, pleaded, "Hold me." He quickly crawled onto my lap. I instinctively wrapped my arms around him like a security blanket. "We'll stay in the room with Chad," I said.

"I'm Dr. K. I am a Pediatric Hematologist/Oncologist. I have looked at Chad's blood work and determined he has leukemia...." Steve and I grasped hands following his pronouncement.

At 3 p.m. on September 25, 1996, my family's life changed forever. I zoned out. His words left me anemic, completely lifeless. I felt blood draining from the top of my head out through my toes. If I had stared at the floor long enough I was sure I would have seen my blood puddle in front of me.

I can't tell you what was spoken following that introductory statement. He spoke for what seemed like an eternity. When he finally finished, we were allowed to ask questions. The game plan was laid out for us, and then we were left alone in a sterile hospital room cradling Chad.

Our next response set the stage for the rest of our unknown journey through the world of childhood cancer. Steve and I, sheltering Chad between us, desperately hugged each other. I looked deeply into Steve's moistened eyes and said, "We're going to go through this with a positive attitude even if it kills us."

We continued hugging each other as we bowed our heads. Once again, we did what we have done so many times in our lives, we prayed to God.

We prayed to the God who is the creator of Chad; the one who knows every hair on his head, and the one who owns

> At 3 p.m. on September 25, 1996, my family's life changed forever. I zoned out.

Chad; the one who loaned us Chad for a season. We prayed to God who is the Father of his perfect son, Jesus Christ, the Great Physician, our rock, our hope, our strength in times of trouble, our tender loving comforter and our Savior!

Releasing Chad to God through prayer was easy to do. We had done it just a year earlier when Chad was three years old. Our family bicycle trip to the Virginia Creeper Trail ended abruptly when Chad, too close to the edge of a fifty foot embankment, toppled end over end with his bicycle and hit a tree with his head. He was airlifted via helicopter to the emergency room.

Although this accident was horrible, it could have been so much worse. Below the tree were massive boulders. Most assuredly Chad's body would have been crushed upon impact had he not been stopped by the tree that God planted for Chad years earlier.

While I yelled for help, Steve and a couple who we had been talking with minutes earlier rappelled down the muddy mountain. Steve reached Chad and began the ascent. He passed Chad up to the man while he pulled himself out of knee high mud.

Hikers and mountain bikers passed me by. Finally, a man stopped. I told him what had happened and that I needed a cell phone to call 911. He handed me his cell phone. I dialed 911 only to hear a busy signal. I tried it again. The call connected. A lady dispatcher informed me that when we did get Chad back up on the trail that we needed to carry him to the entrance of the trail three miles away because the ambulance was too wide to clear the bridge railings. My heart sank. Help was not as close as I had hoped.

I thanked the kind trail traveler and handed the cell phone back to him. I turned away from him for a second to check on Katie and Ryan. I spun back around toward the man only to discover that he had vanished. I can tell you that I do believe in angels and one has a cell phone.

Faint screams pierced the chilly autumn air. Chad was conscious. The man handed Chad to me. A quick triage revealed his left eye was swollen shut and blood was oozing from his nose. Weak cries told of his pain. At that point, my mothering instincts took over. I did what any half crazed mother would do—I sat down in the middle of the trail and began rocking my baby. I thought he was going to die in my arms.

> **Releasing Chad to God through prayer was easy to do. We had done it just a year earlier when Chad was three years old.**

The lady who helped Steve rescue Chad snapped me back to my senses. She said, "You have to get up and start walking toward the entrance of the trail." I obeyed. As we walked, a mass of people assembled around us. Over my right shoulder someone said, "I prayed for him." I said to the lady on my left, "Did you hear that? Someone said, 'I prayed for him.'" She said, "I didn't hear anyone say anything." I knew it was the cell phone angel whispering in my ear.

The crowd was sandwiched by an ambulance approaching in front of us and by a Virginia State Trooper car approaching behind us. Thankfully, the ambulance driver chanced making it through the walking bridges, brushing past the railings.

Upon examination they determined that Chad had head injuries and needed to be airlifted to a hospital about 30 minutes away. Steve, Katie and Ryan rode with the trooper. I rode along with Chad in the ambulance to a cross road where the helicopter awaited in a field.

By this time Chad was slipping in and out of consciousness. Steve and I gave Chad a kiss and said farewell, not really knowing if he would still be alive when we arrived at the hospital.

I sat in the passenger seat of the officer's car with Steve, Katie and Ryan in the back seat. As the trooper prepared to leave the scene I asked him if we could pray. He told us that we could do whatever we needed to do. Steve, Katie, Ryan and I held hands and prayed for Chad. This was the beginning of praying and releasing Chad's life and care into God's hands.

Following the prayer, I sat back in the seat experiencing a calm peace. I, then, asked the officer if I could use his bag cell phone to call the grandparents. He stated that I would have to wait until we got on the interstate because the phone did not have reception in the area where we were. Again, I knew that the angel with the cell phone had a greater reception than any earthly reception man could engineer. I made the dreaded phone calls to the grandparents and to our pastor.

A glance at the speedometer revealed the urgency—115 miles per hour. Apparently, my eyes announced alarm regarding the speed. The officer said that he would just cover up the speedometer because he didn't want to concern me and that he was actually getting ready to speed up. He placed a yellow sticky note over the speedometer and floored the throttle. My head slammed against the headrest. I didn't even want to know how fast we were going.

Following the prayer, I sat back in the seat experiencing a calm peace.

At the hospital, we were ushered into the family waiting room, the room where they tell you your child has died. I slumped into a chair, dropping a bicycle helmet that Chad had put on only seconds before plummeting off the cliff.

To our great relief Chad was in a room being examined. I accompanied him to a facial x-ray that revealed three breaks around his left eye socket. His CAT scan showed more serious injuries. Exhausted, I leaned against the wall only steps away from Chad's side. My eyes shifted from Chad to the physician at the observation window. The concerned look on his face made me sick to my stomach. A few minutes into the scan, Chad began to throw up. The scanning stopped while nurses suctioned him to prevent choking. I asked the physician what he saw on the scan.

This was my first encounter with a physician who missed the "Bedside Manners 101" course.

This was my first encounter with a physician who missed the "Bedside Manners 101" course. With a stone cold face he said, "He has a head injury and we are going to shave his head and cut open his brain to do surgery." I leaned against the wall for physical support as if I had been shot through the heart. My legs numbed. Lethargically I walked beside Chad's stretcher as they returned him to the emergency room.

Once in ICU, a neurosurgeon entered the room. His delightful demeanor was opposite of "Dr. Ice." He said, "I've looked at Chad's CAT scan and determined that we are not going to operate on his brain." Sighs of relief flooded my soul. He explained that the impact on Chad's skull had caused it to overlap in the center, and that as young as Chad was, with time as he grew, the skull too would grow and move back into the proper position. He jovially added, "Mom, you'd better take a picture of Chad's eye because it is a beauty and is going to change colors 50 times before it heals." He put Chad into a drug-induced coma that night to minimize brain activity and the potential for bleeding.

That night I learned how to "pray without ceasing" as 1 Thessalonians 5:17 instructs. Our pastor and Chad's Sunday school teacher came. Few words were spoken. We prayed together and we prayed individually. Only the beeping of the monitors filled the silent room.

The next morning Chad awoke asking for french fries. He was moved into a guarded pediatric room. That afternoon his left eye peeked through a swollen and badly bruised eyelid.

The hospital guard who was on duty when we arrived delivered Chad's forgotten bicycle helmet. Upon inspection I shook to discover a puncture hole in the helmet. It looked as though someone had driven a spike into it. Chad had struck something knife sharp during his drop down the cliff or in his impact with the tree. Whatever it was, God had protected him from a life-ending blow.

The next day Chad was released with a concussion and three breaks around his eye-socket but no permanent damage to his vision. His two-week follow-up showed the skull already moving back into its normal position.

The weeks following the accident were trying to say the least. The headaches that Chad suffered left him running violently around the house in circles. The only calming time was when he rode in the car.

One particular night, Steve was working late and Chad was running crazy. I called Steve to let him know that he could work as long as he needed to but that Chad and I were going driving around. I told Steve that we might drive to Knoxville and back (about a five hour trip). I had to have some peace. This was my first experience of being the caregiver of a child with a serious illness/accident.

Then just over a year later I was put into the care-giving role of a seriously ill child. This "rehearsal," if you will, helped me to know exactly what I needed to do when Chad was diagnosed at age four with leukemia—PRAY.

This "rehearsal," if you will, helped me to know exactly what I needed to do when Chad was diagnosed at age four with leukemia—PRAY.

Friends, that was ten years ago. God has been with me every step of this journey called life. I am nothing without him. I could not have done this on my own strength. Prayers continue to carry me. Be assured, when asked, he will do the same for you.

Hugs and Prayers,
Rita

Caring with TLC

Finding Hope to Cope Together

"'For where two or three come together in my name, there am I with them.'"

—Jesus (Matthew 18:20)

Welcome & Purpose

Welcome to the TLC For Parents support group. The purpose of the group is:

to share the love, grace, and mercy of Christ Jesus with each other by sharing and bearing each other's burdens, expressing our love and care for one another, and encouraging each other so that we might find hope to cope while caring for our seriously ill child.

Opening Prayer

Dear God who comforts parents of seriously ill children and gives us hope and strength to cope, thank you for drawing each one of us together here and now. Lord Jesus, we have come together in your name and know that you are here with us as you promised. Lift our spirits and heal our broken hearts! Let your love, mercy, grace, hope and truth guide us as we comfort and encourage one another in your name. Amen.

Hanging On & Hanging Out

CarePoint believes that "The greatest untapped source of healing in the world is a word of encouragement spoken by one believer to another."

According to my Senior Pastor, Ben Cachiaras, there are two vital relationships in life—hanging on and hanging out.

The first, hanging on, is our relationship with God based on trust in Jesus Christ.

The second vital relationship in life is hanging out. This involves deep, vital fellowship with other Christian followers. Fellowship comes from the Greek word *koinonia*. That word represents sharing. Ben says it best, "When we hang out together it helps us hang on."

Ben says it best, "When we hang out together it helps us hang on."

Getting Started

❶ Since the heart of a small group is interaction, take a moment to introduce yourself to everyone. Share something about yourself with the group. (In the space below you may want to jot a note or two as each member shares.)

_____

_____

_____

_____

_____

Our Group Covenant

This group is a covenant group. Covenants help us to build trust, share openly, and love and care for each other on the hills and in the valleys of our lives. Agreeing to a covenant for our group at the outset is important. Your group shepherd will provide you with a sample covenant. As a group you can do with it as you will: adopt it as it is, adopt it and adapt it, or scrap it and draft your own from scratch.

TLC Truth

Speaking truth out of our mouth is an excellent avenue to travel as we seek God's truth in caring for ourselves, for our family and for our seriously ill child.

Weekly, in each week's homework, and as a foundation for the next week's study, we will highlight a "TLC Truth." This workbook contains 10 truths to speak aloud daily. Satan desires to destroy our relationship with God. He will do that in any way possible. Speaking truth out of our mouth is an excellent avenue to travel as we seek God's truth in caring for ourselves, for our family and for our seriously ill child.

In John 8:31-32 Jesus told the Jews who believed in him, "If you hold to my teaching, you are really my disciples. Then you will know the truth, and the truth will set you free." Although the mind will likely scoff at these Truths, covet them, speak them, and think about them! This is an activity that can help set you free!

TLC Truth

#1: God cares about my needs.

How Jesus Ministered to the Seriously Ill and Their Parents

He Touched them. He Listened to them. He had Compassion on them. Someone volunteer to read Mark 5:22-24, 35-43, the story of a man with a seriously ill child. As you read, note where Jesus uses touch, listens and shows compassion.

> *Then one of the synagogue rulers, named Jairus, came there. Seeing Jesus, he fell at his feet and pleaded earnestly with him, "My little daughter is dying. Please come and put your hands on her so that she will be healed and live." So Jesus went with him.*
>
> *While Jesus was still speaking, some men came from the house of Jairus, the synagogue ruler. "Your daughter is dead," they said. "Why bother the teacher any more?"*
>
> *Ignoring what they said, Jesus told the synagogue ruler, "Don't be afraid; just believe."*
>
> *He did not let anyone follow him except Peter, James and John the brother of James. When they came to the home of the synagogue ruler, Jesus saw a commotion, with people crying and wailing loudly.*
>
> *He went in and said to them, "Why all this commotion and wailing? The child is not dead but asleep." But they laughed at him.*
>
> *After he put them all out, he took the child's father and mother and the disciples who were with him, and went in where the child was. He took her by the hand and said to her, "Talitha koum!" (which means, "Little girl, I say to you, get up!"). Immediately the girl stood up and walked around (she was twelve years old). At this they were completely astonished. He gave strict orders not to let anyone know about this, and told them to give her something to eat.*

Many times, Jesus used touch in ways that brought healing to the sick, as we see in the previous example. There were also times when Jesus used touch to alleviate fear, which we may commonly feel in caring for a seriously ill child. Someone volunteer to read this passage from Matthew 17:1-8.

> *After six days Jesus took with him Peter, James and John the brother of James, and led them up a high mountain by themselves. There he was transfigured before them. His face shone like the sun, and his clothes became as white as the light. Just then there appeared before them Moses and Elijah, talking with Jesus.*
>
> *Peter said to Jesus, "Lord, it is good for us to be here. If you wish, I will put up three shelters—one for you, one for Moses and one for Elijah."*
>
> *While he was still speaking, a bright cloud enveloped them, and a voice from the cloud said, "This is my Son, whom I love; with him I am well pleased. Listen to him!"*
>
> *When the disciples heard this, they fell facedown to the ground, terrified. But Jesus came and touched them. "Get up," he said. "Don't be afraid." When they looked up, they saw no one except Jesus.*

❷ Are there ways you've sensed the comforting touch of God as you've cared for your child? Explain.

_____

_____

_____

_____

_____

❸ Has the Lord brought comforting touch to you through someone else? Talk about your experience.

_____

_____

_____

_____

_____

Jesus wants to listen to your heart and your emotions.

Jesus wants to listen to your heart and your emotions. He wants to hear your pain, your joy; he wants you to tell him about your exhaustion, your shattered dreams, and the hope you're holding onto.

❹ Have you been able to share your heart and your emotions with the Lord? To what extent? If not, what do you think keeps you from doing this?

_____

_____

_____

_____

_____

Jesus has a heart of compassion toward those who are hurting and weary from caring for others.

❺ Are there ways the Lord has shown his compassion toward you? Explain.

_____

_____

_____

_____

_____

Jesus demonstrated by example what the seriously ill and their parents want and need most: TLC. We need a gentle Touch to comfort, a Listening ear to sound upon and a Compassionate heart to sympathize.

> Jesus demonstrated by example what the seriously ill and their parents want and need most: TLC.

❻ List here ways you can begin to support each other with TLC (Touch, a Listening ear and Compassion). Share your own TLC needs with the group.

_____

_____

_____

_____

Reflection & Encouragement

"My only concern is that unless they (caregivers) realize that self-care is the first job for any caregiver, any bit of advice offered may not be acted upon. And caring for ourselves may be the most fearless act of care giving any of us can commit. After all, as my friend Chuck says, 'Even Jesus didn't carry the cross the entire way alone.'"

—Gary Barg

Strength for the Week

Share prayer requests. List them below and pray for these members and their requests throughout the week.

_____

_____

_____

_____

_____

Closing Prayer

Dear Lord, thank you for drawing us together in fellowship. Lift our spirits and give us hope to cope, even now at the outset of our loving Christian fellowship. We know that all good things come from above, and we thank you for caring for us and for our children even more than we do. Draw us close to you and to each other in the days to come. In Jesus' name we pray. Amen.

Week 1 Memory Verse

"Though one may be overpowered, two can defend themselves. A cord of three strands is not quickly broken." (Ecclesiastes 4:12)

Homework

❶ Daily read **TLC Truth #2**: Emotions are a gift from God to be appropriately expressed not suppressed.

❷ Read *Introduction & Encouragement* section (beginning on page 11).

❸ Read *Facts & Figures: Parents of Children with Serious Illnesses* (beginning on page 15).

❹ Read *Rita's Story* (beginning on page 17).

❺ Read devotional entries 1-5 (beginning on page 103).

❻ Complete Week 2 in preparation for next week's group.

Caring for the Caregiver Emotionally
Living Beyond Your Feelings

"In my anguish I cried to the Lord, and he answered by setting me free. The Lord is with me; I will not be afraid."
—Psalm 118:5-6

Opening Prayer

Dear God, we thank you for gifting us with emotions. Help us to live beyond our feelings by appropriately expressing our emotions instead of suppressing them. Teach us to express our emotions to you. In Jesus' name we pray. Amen.

TLC Truth

#2: Emotions are a gift from God to be appropriately expressed not suppressed.

Devotional Questions

Emotions—Straighten Out the Roller Coaster Ride

❶ What emotions do you feel? Don't stop to think about them just write them down quickly.

_____

_____

_____

_____

❷ After reading this devotional, how do you think God feels about your emotions?

_____

_____

_____

_____

_____

❸ Based on Psalm 46:10, how does God want you to respond to your emotions?

_____

_____

_____

_____

_____

❹ Have you handed over your most precious ornament to Jesus to hold onto while you're on this emotional roller coaster ride?

_____

_____

_____

_____

_____

The Diagnosis—Why?

❺ Have you asked God, "Why?" If so, how do you sense God answering your question?

_____

_____

_____

_____

6 God doesn't always answer us as we'd like. Have you moved past or come to peaceful terms with your question of "Why?"

_____

_____

_____

_____

_____

7 Various emotional stages are normal: denial, isolation or loneliness, fear, worry, guilt, anger, bargaining, depression, acceptance, and hope are emotions we may experience in any order and repeatedly. Which of these emotional stages have you experienced?

_____

_____

_____

_____

_____

8 Have you aimed your emotions at someone else instead of God? If so, at whom?

_____

_____

_____

_____

9 Do you need to ask or have you asked for forgiveness from that person? If so, contact that person today asking for forgiveness.

_____

_____

_____

_____

_____

The Blame Game—How?

10 Have you been playing a blame game? If so, which blame game(s) have you been playing?

_____

_____

_____

_____

_____

11 Ask for forgiveness from that person and from God. Choose today to stop playing the blame game and to get in the game of real life where there is no condemnation by Jesus but only sweet time to magnify God for all of his blessings and mercies.

_____

_____

_____

_____

12 According to John 9:3, what might God's purpose be in your circumstances?

_____

_____

_____

_____

_____

Shattered Dreams—Grieving the Child Who Will Not Exist

13 Have you allowed yourself to grieve for the child that
will not exist? If so, how did you grieve?

_____

_____

_____

_____

_____

14 If you have not worked through the initial grieving process for the child that will not exist answer the following
question: Name some activities that your child may not
get to experience due to his illness, injury or birth defect?

_____

_____

_____

_____

_____

15 If you have worked through the initial grieving process,
jot down remembrances of that time and the emotions
you felt and how God comforted you throughout the
process.

_____

_____

_____

_____

_____

16 React to the quote from the fictional character Larkspur
Summerville in this reading section. In what ways do
you long for God to comfort you?

_____

_____

_____

_____

_____

17 In what ways does Jeremiah 29:11 speak to you about your needs and longings?

_____

_____

_____

_____

_____

If—Today Our Child is Living with (fill in your child's illness, injury or birth defect)

18 Describe an "If Only" memory you wish you could change.

_____

_____

_____

_____

_____

19 Describe a "What If" worry you have about the future.

_____

_____

_____

_____

_____

Pray and ask God to help you change your thinking about the past, present and future.

Reflection & Encouragement

"If you paint in your mind a picture of bright and happy expectations, you put yourself into a condition conducive to your goal."

—Norman Vincent Peale

"Most folks are about as happy as they make up their minds to be."

—Abraham Lincoln

Strength for the Week

Share prayer requests. List them below and pray for these members and their requests throughout the week.

_____

_____

_____

_____

_____

Closing Prayer

Dear Lord, thank you for our God given emotions. Help us to learn from Jesus' example to appropriately express our emotions and not to suppress them. Also, help us to turn to you as an outlet to express our emotions being assured that you can handle every emotion we feel. In Jesus' name. Amen.

Week 2 Memory Verse

"Cast all your anxiety on him because he cares for you." (1 Peter 5:7)

Homework

❶ Daily read **TLC Truth #3**: Faith in God can transform me from fearful to fearless.

❷ Read devotional entries 6-10 (beginning on page 111).

❸ Complete Week 3 in preparation for next week's group.

Caring for the Caregiver Spiritually
Experiencing an Intimate Relationship with God

"Cast your cares on the Lord and he will sustain you; he will never let the righteous fall."

—Psalm 55:22

Opening Prayer

Dear Lord, thank you for loving us and giving us hope, eternal hope, that all will be well. For you have saved us from our sins and are the Light that shines in all the dark places of our hearts and our world. Deliver us from evil and help us resist the enemy by the power of the cross! In Jesus' name we pray. Amen.

TLC Truth

#3 Faith in God can transform me from fearful to fearless.

Devotional Questions

Fear of Death—Facing our Greatest Fear

❶ Did you make a commitment to Christ or a re-commitment you would like to share with the group?

_____

_____

_____

_____

_____

Fear and Faith—From Fearful to Fearless

❷ Describe a time when you felt inadequate to care for your child.

_____

_____

_____

_____

_____

❸ React to the statement, "The truth is that God doesn't call the qualified. God qualifies the called." Talk about how this helps move you from fearful to fearless.

_____

_____

_____

_____

_____

❹ What examples can you share about God's provision despite your feelings of inadequacy?

_____

_____

_____

_____

_____

Prayer—The Most Powerful Medicine

❺ Have you established a prayer relay team? If yes, what is the person's name that heads it up? This week send that person a thank you note expressing your gratitude for his or her faithful servant's heart.

_____

_____

_____

_____

_____

❻ If you have not already established a prayer relay team
for your family, pray about whom God would have you
ask to head the team up. When God brings a person to
mind contact the person asking him or her to head up
the prayer relay team on your family's behalf.

_____

_____

_____

_____

God's Promises in the Bible—At the Least, Comfort; At the Best, Healing

❼ Pray asking God to speak to you as you read the scripture references listed in my friend's note. Next, steal
away to a quiet place. Look up and meditate on each
verse. Write the verse that gives you the greatest comfort.

_____

_____

_____

_____

Loneliness—Where is God?

❽ Has there been a time during your child's illness when
you experienced feelings of loneliness or depression? Describe that time.

_____

_____

_____

_____

_____

9 In what ways did you find relief and/or comfort?

_____

_____

_____

_____

_____

10 Did you reach out to others for support? Do you need that type of support at this time? Express your heart and needs to others (possibly in this group) who can pray for you, support you, listen to your heart and help carry your burden (Galatians 6:2).

_____

_____

_____

_____

_____

11 Did you seek or do you need to seek help from a doctor? If yes, I encourage you to take that step by scheduling an appointment today.

_____

_____

_____

_____

_____

Certainly, continue to seek the Lord who hears and cares deeply for the lonely. Psalm 55:16-17 says, "But I call to God, and the Lord saves me. Evening, morning and noon I cry out in distress, and he hears my voice."

Are you at Peace with God?

Try as we may, if we have anything in our conscience that is contrary to God, we will not be able to experience true peace in our hearts.

We need to have peace with God before we can experience true lasting peace that conquers anxiety. All of us have a God-shaped vacuum; we were created to experience a relationship with him. The only way this relationship with our Heavenly Father can occur is through his son, Jesus Christ (John 14:6 "I am the way, the truth and the life. No one comes to the Father except through me").

So, first and foremost, consider if you are absolutely certain that you have a relationship with God through Jesus Christ. If you have any doubt that you have accepted what Jesus did on the cross personally for your sins, and if you're not one hundred percent sure if you have received his free gift of eternal life, this is where to start to experience true peace. If you will but pray a simple prayer like this and mean it in your heart, God has promised to save you.

> *Dear Lord, I acknowledge that I have not followed your way. I ask now for you to forgive me of all my sin. I believe that you willingly died on the cross for my sins, rose again, and reign as my Savior; thank you that I am now pure in your sight because of what Jesus did on the cross for me. You love me like no other, and desire to come into my life. I accept your gift of salvation. Guide me, Lord, and grant me peace. Thank you. In Jesus' name. Amen.*

If you just prayed this prayer of salvation for the first time, all of heaven is rejoicing! God has saved you from your sin; he loves you and is with you! He has come into your life and will never leave you (Hebrews 13:5). This is the most crucial decision you can make because not only will your new relationship with Christ influence your life on earth, but it will also assure you of eternal life (1 John 5:12). Christianity is not about religion; it's a growing relationship with the living God who longs to fellowship with us.

As a believer in Christ, you can deepen your relationship with him through:

- Prayer (Psalm 50:15; Matthew 6:5-13; 1 Thessalonians 5:17)

- Praise and worship (Psalm 50:23; James 4:8)

- Bible study (Psalm 119:11; 2 Timothy 3:15-17)

We need to have peace with God before we can experience true lasting peace that conquers anxiety.

- Serving others (Matthew 25:34-46)
- Spending time with other believers (Hebrews 10:25)

You may not be ready to take this step to pray the prayer. It's not about just saying the words with your mouth. It's the faith that matters. Take time if you need to search your heart and soul. Ask questions. Ponder the answers. Seek God for understanding. Christ is knocking at your heart, but you're the only one who can decide if you want to open the door to let him in.

"Yet to all who received him, to those who believed in his name, he gave the right to become children of God" (John 1:12).

If you have made a decision to accept Christ as your personal Lord and Savior for the first time, consider telling the other members of the group so they can celebrate with you. Ask them to share their "stories" with you of how they came to know Jesus. Please jot me an e-mail so that I may rejoice with you and pray for you.

Reflection & Encouragement

"He who has faith has hope; and he who has hope has everything."

—Ancient Proverb

"You don't have to be superhuman or even super-spiritual to parent a child through crisis. You simply have to value your child and provide the tools she needs. Your compassionate presence, loving care, and steady guidance are critical to your child making it through unscarred. All children need certain expressions of this love... But the specific ways you meet these needs are up to God and you."

—Karen Dockrey

Strength for the Week

Share praises and prayer requests. List them below and pray for these members and their requests throughout the week.

_____

_____

_____

_____

_____

Closing Prayer

Dear Lord, maker of heaven and earth and Lord of all, thank you for giving us the truth of your word to resist the enemy and his hosts! Help us each day to realize the attacks of the devil and to resist them through the power of your word. Lift our spirits with your hope! And keep us in the truth that you and your boundless light and love are with us even in the dark valleys of life. In Jesus' name we pray. Amen.

Week 3 Memory Verse

"Submit yourselves, then, to God. Resist the devil, and he will flee from you. Come near to God and he will come near to you." (James 4:7-8a)

Homework

❶ Daily read **TLC Truth #4**: My body is a temple of the Holy Spirit, designed to bring honor to God.

❷ Read devotional entries 11-15 (beginning on page 118).

❸ Complete Week 4 in preparation for next week's group.

Caring for the Caregiver Physically

Stress Management Tools

"Do you not know that your body is a temple of the Holy Spirit, who is in you, whom you have received from God? You are not your own; you were bought at a price. Therefore honor God with your body."

— *1 Corinthians 6:19-20*

Opening Prayer

Dear Lord, thank you for creating us in your image. We praise you that you knit us together in our mother's womb. We praise you because we are fearfully and wonderfully made. Your works are wonderful. Help us to be good stewards of the bodies you have blessed us with. In Jesus' name we pray. Amen.

TLC Truth

#4: My body is a temple of the Holy Spirit, designed to bring honor to God.

Devotional Questions

Rest—A Gift from God

❶ What despairing thoughts do you need to acknowledge and release to God?

_____

_____

_____

_____

_____

2 What are your hopeful thoughts?

_____

_____

_____

_____

_____

3 Reflect on the statement "When despairing thoughts creep into our minds, turn to God asking him to quiet our minds and to direct our thoughts to focus on the present and the blessings we have close at hand…." Share about how this statement impacts you.

_____

_____

_____

_____

_____

4 This week name one strategy you will use to rest.

_____

_____

_____

_____

Nutrition and Exercise—Loving Ourselves

5 List practical things you can do for your health. (It may be to make an appointment for a physical, a mammogram, an annual pap smear, a dental visit, or to begin walking, eating healthier, etc.)

_____

_____

_____

_____

_____

Real Friends / Support Groups—It's Okay to Cry

❻ Describe a way that God has provided support for you through another person.

_____

_____

_____

_____

_____

❼ Call a TLC group member that God puts on your heart. They need you. Take time to listen. Ask them how you can specifically pray for them; write it below and pray.

_____

_____

_____

_____

Attitude of Gratitude—"Someone's not Happy but We are."

❽ Think of three people you can thank for something they have done in your life. List those people and then write a note card of thanks or phone them to express your gratitude for what they did for you.

_____

_____

_____

_____

Perseverance / Admit Our Weaknesses—Strength for the Day / Ask for Help

9 In what ways have others reached out to help you?

_____

_____

_____

_____

_____

10 Who has made an offer of help that you have not yet accepted?

_____

_____

_____

_____

_____

11 Contact those people thanking them and accepting their offers.

_____

_____

_____

_____

_____

> The enemy whispers that we do not have time to take care of ourselves because we are busy caring for our child.

The Enemy & Caring for the Caregiver Physically

This week as we turn our thoughts toward caring for ourselves we want to examine the enemy's lies. The enemy whispers that we do not have time to take care of ourselves because we are busy caring for our child. We feel deprived. Resentment sets in. Then we have a bad attitude. Finally, we look at life as a burden instead of a blessing.

God's word, on the contrary, says that as a child of God we are temples of the Holy Spirit and as such we are to honor God with our bodies. This is God's prescription of how to care for ourselves. We must choose to believe and obey God on this issue. He loves us and wants only his best for us. Physical pain and suffering can be avoided by following God's prescription plan for our health.

Reflection & Encouragement

"Compassion is the keen awareness of the interdependence of all things."

—Thomas Merton

"Reflect upon your present blessings—of which every man has many—not on your past misfortunes, of which all men have some."

—Charles Dickens

Strength for the Week

Share praises and prayer requests. List them below and pray for these members and their requests throughout the week.

_____

_____

_____

_____

_____

Closing Prayer

Dear Lord, we praise you because we are fearfully and wonderfully made by you. Your works are wonderful. Help us daily identify the attacks of the devil and to resist them through the power of your word. Please reveal your plan for our physical bodies that you have bought with a price through Jesus' blood. Help us to honor you with our bodies that are a temple of the Holy Spirit. In Jesus' name we pray. Amen.

Week 4 Memory Verse

"Do you not know that your body is a temple of the Holy Spirit, who is in you, whom you have received from God? You are not your own; you were bought at a price. Therefore honor God with your body." (1 Corinthians 6:19-20)

Homework

❶ Daily read **TLC Truth** **#5**: Families are one of God's greatest treasures on earth to be cherished and protected during the storm.

❷ Read devotional entries 16-19 (beginning on page 143).

❸ Complete Week 5 in preparation for next week's group.

Caring for the Clan Emotionally & Spiritually
Caring for Those We Love the Most

"'Therefore everyone who hears these words of mine and puts them into practice is like a wise man who built his house on the rock. The rain came down, the streams rose, and the winds blew and beat against that house; yet it did not fall, because it had its foundation on the rock.'"

—Matthew 7:25-26

Opening Prayer

Father God, we thank you for your perfect design of the family. We thank you for our families you have blessed us with. They are a gift from you. Please give us wisdom and knowledge of how to care for those we love most who are also traveling on this journey with us and who are hurting too. Bless them and hold them close to you. In Jesus' name we pray. Amen.

TLC Truth

#5: Families are one of God's greatest treasures on earth to be cherished and protected during the storm.

Devotional Questions

The Diagnosis—Telling Family Members

❶ Describe how you told family members about your child's diagnosis, and describe their responses.

_____

_____

_____

_____

_____

❷ In what ways has the news bonded or distanced relation-ships?

_____

_____

_____

_____

_____

Father / Mother—Unite for the Common Cause

❸ In your situation, are both the father and the mother in-volved in caring for the child?

_____

_____

_____

_____

_____

❹ If both of you are involved, what strengths do you see each of you offering? (Express gratefulness for the other's strengths and involvement.)

_____

_____

_____

_____

_____

❺ If one parent is uninvolved or minimally involved, what is one step you can take to encourage the other parent to

be present in the seriously ill child's life? (Carefully consider what may be inhibiting his or her involvement, e.g.,
fear, illness, Satan's lies, etc.)

_____

_____

_____

_____

_____

The Other Children—What about us?

❻ Have you noticed changes in the other child(ren)'s behavior since the diagnosis of your child?

_____

_____

_____

_____

_____

❼ If so, what changes have caught your attention as being
unusual for that child?

_____

_____

_____

_____

_____

Determine a time this week to have some one-on-one time
with each child. Play is a wonderful time for a child's
thoughts to spill out in a carefree manner. Drawing also pro-
motes thoughts to silently spill onto paper. Leading questions
lend to discussion. Also, bedtime is a great time when children relax and share thoughts. I still enjoy scratching my children's backs and listening as they share their thoughts and
concerns. There's nothing like a good back scratching to help
someone let her guard down and share her heart.

Determine a time this week to have some one-on-one time with each child. Play is a wonderful time for a child's thoughts to spill out in a carefree manner.

Home Sweet Home—There's No Place Like Home

8 Could you relate to feeling like an Oreo cookie? Explain.

_____

_____

_____

_____

_____

9 What "ground rules" or boundaries have you set up, or can you set up, to help reduce stress?

_____

_____

_____

_____

_____

10 In what ways have you accepted, or can you accept, the help (esp. in the areas of their gifts and talents) of well-meaning friends?

_____

_____

_____

_____

_____

11 Since your family routine has been disrupted, list one item you would like to add to your new family routine.

_____

_____

_____

_____

_____

⓬ List one item you do not want to put back onto your family calendar.

_____

_____

_____

_____

_____

Caring for the Clan Emotionally and Spiritually

This week we focus on our family members. All too often we submerge ourselves with caring for our seriously ill child while our spouse and other children received the left over crumbs of our time and attention. They suffer in silence. Feelings of neglect brew and eventually boil over. It is critical to our family's life that we set up the dynamics for a family of inclusion not exclusion.

⓭ Go around the room and share struggles you face in caring for your clan. (Examples may include lack of time, distance away from home, etc.)

_____

_____

_____

_____

_____

All too often we submerge ourselves with caring for our seriously ill child while our spouse and other children received the left over crumbs of our time and attention.

We find comfort knowing that we all struggle in this area. The key to survival is relying on God to reveal the needs of family members. There are always more things we could do. This is another lie of Satan's—that we aren't doing everything we could in caring for the clan while caring for the seriously ill child. God's truth is that we must rely on him to quicken our mind for each family member's need.

Reflection & Encouragement

"Cancer is not a solo act. The entire family unit is affected in some way, great or small."
—Nancy Brown

Strength for the Week

Share praises and prayer requests. List them below and pray for these members and their requests throughout the week.

_____

_____

_____

_____

_____

Closing Prayer

Father God, we thank you for the gift of family. Please give us wisdom and knowledge of exactly what you would have us do for each family member. Help us to love with your love. We thank you for this group, our second family, and their love, support and prayers. In Jesus' name we pray. Amen.

Week 5 Memory Verse

"I can do everything through him who gives me strength." (Philippians 4:13)

Homework

❶ Daily read **TLC Truth #6**: Humans are God's only creation that worries.

❷ Read devotional entries 20-21 (beginning on page 133). There are fewer devotions this week so that we can roll up our sleeves to work on the finances.

❸ Complete Week 6 in preparation for next week's group.

Caring for the Clan Physically

Facing Finances & Insurance

"And my God will meet all your needs according to his glorious riches in Christ Jesus."

—*Philippians 4:19*

Opening Prayer

Father God, we are reminded of Psalm 109:22 where David cried out to you, saying, "For I am poor and needy, and my heart is wounded within me." Father we confess that in caring for a seriously ill child we have also faced great financial burdens. As we look at this area of our lives from the biblical perspective, help us to trust in you to meet all of our needs according to your glorious riches in Jesus Christ. In Jesus' name we pray. Amen.

TLC Truth

#6: Humans are God's only creation that worries.

Devotional Questions

Financial Needs—Confess and Swallow Our Pride

❶ What financial burdens have you encountered through your child's illness?

_____

_____

_____

_____

❷ Do you sense a need for financial help?

_____

_____

_____

_____

_____

❸ First, pray and ask God how he wants to provide for you?

_____

_____

_____

_____

_____

❹ Besides informing those in your group, consider if there is someone with whom God would have you share your financial need. Then, go to that person asking for help. Chances are that God has already put you on that person's heart. Remember he goes before us.

_____

_____

_____

_____

_____

❺ Are there ways in which you are resistant to help? If so, consider if God would have you humble yourself to receive help?

_____

_____

_____

_____

_____

Insurance—Learn to Play the Game

❻ Describe how you could relate to Julie Gordon's "What did you do all day?"

_____

_____

_____

_____

❼ You have much to do. Pray asking for God's help as you make phone calls. Set aside time to make any needed phone calls to medical providers or insurance. Ask God to make the fruit of the Spirit abound in your life.

Caring for the Clan Physically—Facing Finances & Insurance

One of the biggest ways we care for our clan is by working to put a roof over their heads, food on the table and clothes on their backs.

In the beginning of caring for our child, people asked us if we need anything, meals or money. We always replied, "No. No. We think our insurance is going to do pretty well in paying the medical bills."

Perhaps the medical insurance is pretty good at paying the bills, yet a balance or co-pay is owed. Maybe there's a deductible that must be met before insurance begins paying. Each service rendered has a small balance but when lumped into the entire amount owed it adds up.

Doctor K asked me, "Do you work?" "Yes, I work part-time," I replied. "You don't anymore," was his reply. Typically, parents of a child with a serious illness are forced to make the decision that one parent, usually the mother, will quit the job or at least take a leave of absence for a while, to care for the needs of the child.

A single parent is either forced to attempt to go back to work with the help of friends and relatives covering the bases of doctor appointments, treatments, and caring for the child

> In the beginning of caring for our child, people asked us if we need anything, meals or money. We always replied, "No...."

> Then the enemy sends the spirit of fear and worry to our doorstep. If we allow this visitor to enter, we eventually become overwhelmed and meet our breaking point.

at home, or is forced to quit his or her current job, take an extended leave of absence without pay, or pursue a new vocation that allows work to be done from home. Either choice is a difficult decision.

When medical bills start coming in, what seemed to be manageable in the beginning grows to be unbearable. Then the enemy sends the spirit of fear and worry to our doorstep. If we allow this visitor to enter, we eventually become overwhelmed and meet our breaking point. It is not God's design for us to get to the point of breaking. We get ourselves to the point of breaking by taking on worry that God never intended for us. God, though, patiently waits for his children to ask for help. Matthew 6:28-34 offers comfort in knowing that our loving God knows our needs and has a plan to provide even when we can't see the answer or the way.

God never intended for us to carry the financial burden alone. Larry Burkett's book *Hope When It Hurts: A Personal Testimony of How to Deal with the Impact of Cancer* (particularly Chapter Eleven, "What to Do When Your Money Runs Out") provides a biblical financial model to follow in handling the extra expenses that come with having a child with a serious illness. Burkett was also affiliated with Crown Financial Ministries before his death in 2003 following his battle with cancer. The Crown website (www.crown.org) offers a wealth of information on finances, debt, and money management.

Two Attitudes to Keep When The Bills Mount Up

1. Be Honest with Your Doctors, Hospitals, and Church Family.

Lay out your situation up front, even before surgery or treatment, especially if you don't have insurance. Tell the provider that you don't have the money to pay the costs. Public hospitals that receive government funds are required by law to treat you, so they can't turn you away. Being honest enhances your integrity. There may be a Christian doctor who will provide the services for free.

2. God is in Control Even When You Are Not

Mounting medical bills, coupled with health uncertainties of the future, may leave you in a tailspin, wondering if things will ever settle down again. But no matter how out of control things seem to you, remember that God has not forgotten you. In Matthew 28, Jesus declared that all authority in heaven and on earth belonged to him. In faith, let him exercise his power in your life when things seem so out of control.

Where to Find Help

You Are Responsible For Doing What You Can

The first responsibility we have as children of God is to take responsibility for what we can pay. Galatians 6:5 tells us that each one should carry his own load.

Approach Your Extended Family

Next, when we have paid all that we are capable of paying we openly express needs to our family members. 1 Timothy 5:4 instructs that children and grandchildren of widows are "to put their religion into practice by caring for their own family and so repaying their parents and grandparents, for this is pleasing to God."

Seek Assistance from Your Church Family

There will be times when Christians in need should approach their church families for financial assistance. That's completely biblical, and the precedent is seen clearly in scripture. Your first thoughts may be that of standing outside the pastor's office with stacks of medical bills in hand, feeling like a beggar. That's our pride showing through. Just because some abuse the generosity of others does not make sharing a need with your church wrong.

> There will be times when Christians in need should approach their church families for financial assistance.

What to Do When the Money Runs Out

1. Don't Worry

What if no one steps up to the plate after you make your needs known? The fundamental principle to keep in mind is, don't worry. Worry is taking on a responsibility that belongs to God. God's desire is for you to do what's within your ability to do and then be at peace.

2. Liquidate Your Assets

If you have an emergency fund, your situation may be such an emergency. As far as selling your home goes. Larry Burkett's advice is if you took the treatment and the provider knew in advance that you weren't going to be able to pay for it, then virtually no doctor or hospital is going to ask you to sell your home to pay bills. He makes a wonderful point by saying that often the situation is taxing enough on finances; being homeless may be too much to bear. He does caution about jumping into bankruptcy too quickly as a way out.

3. If You Have to Consider Bankruptcy

Bankruptcy should be a last resort, not a first option. Larry suggests considering filing for bankruptcy protection, however, if the mental health of you or your spouse is of serious concern, if creditors attempt to take hold of all of your assets to the exclusion of all others, or if they place pressure on you to break laws or engage in illegal or immoral behavior.

God has the resources to meet all of our needs. He owns everything in heaven and earth. A few extra medical bills are just small change to him. He holds out his hands waiting for us to give him these worries and invite him to make a way to meet these needs.

> God has the resources to meet all of our needs. He owns everything in heaven and earth.

Reflection & Encouragement

"When it comes down to it, if you don't have good health insurance, you're going to be obligated for thousands of dollars of expenses. The bottom line is, do the best you can do, as unto the Lord, and trust God. Walk in peace. God doesn't expect you to do things you cannot do, only the things that are within the realm of possibility as you trust him."

—Larry Burkett

Strength for the Week

Share praises and prayer requests. List them below and pray for these members and their requests throughout the week.

_____

_____

_____

_____

_____

Closing Prayer

Father God, thank you for your instruction about worry. Help us turn over our mounting bills and financial needs to you. Help us to apply biblical financial concepts. We trust you to provide for all of our needs through your glorious riches in Jesus Christ in whose name we pray. Amen.

Week 6 Memory Verse

"But seek first his kingdom and his righteous-
ness, and all these things will be given to you as
well." (Matthew 6:33)

Homework

❶ Daily read **TLC Truth** #7: God calls parents to be cheerleaders for their children by encouraging them, comforting them and urging them to live lives worthy of God.
(from 1 Thessalonians 2:12)

❷ Read devotional entries 22-26 (beginning on page 160).

❸ Complete Week 7 in preparation for next week's group.

Caring for the Seriously Ill Child Emotionally

Cheering Him on to Victory

"...turning your ear to wisdom and applying your heart to understanding, and if you call out for insight and cry aloud for understanding, and if you look for it as for silver and search for it as for hidden treasure, then you will understand the fear of the Lord and find the knowledge of God."

—*Proverbs 2:2-5*

Opening Prayer

Father God, as we focus on how to care for our child emotionally, we claim your promise in Proverbs 2:4-5 that tells us if we search for wisdom, insight and understanding like treasure you will be faithful to us and we will find your knowledge. Help us be an encouragement and support to one another as we share our successes and lessons learned in helping our child emotionally. In Jesus' name we pray. Amen.

TLC Truth

#7: God calls parents to be cheerleaders for their children by encouraging them, comforting them and urging them to live lives worthy of God. (from 1 Thessalonians 2:12)

Devotional Questions

The Diagnosis—What Do We Tell Our Child?

❶ Recount how your child learned of his life-threatening illness.

_____

_____

_____

_____

_____

② Do you struggle or have you struggled with openly communicating with your child? Why do you think that is?

_____

_____

_____

_____

③ Do you sense that your child feels completely free to share his feelings with you? If not, consider ways in which you can help him feel more comfortable sharing with you. Ask group members for suggestions.

_____

_____

_____

_____

④ Describe one open communication strategy you use with your child.

_____

_____

_____

_____

The Prognosis—I Might Die. If I Die Will You Go with Me?

5 Are you prepared to answer your child's questions about death and dying?

_____

_____

_____

_____

_____

6 If you have not yet formulated an answer to your child's questions about death and dying, think about your potential response. Write it here.

_____

_____

_____

_____

_____

7 If your child has not yet asked you about death and dying, has your child made comments, perhaps written something, made something, or drawn a picture that causes you to believe he is thinking about death and would like to talk about it but is not sure what to say or ask?

_____

_____

_____

_____

_____

8 If so, how might you take the next step in talking with your child about death and dying?

_____

_____

_____

_____

_____

Attitude with a Capital A—The Strong Willed Child Takes on Life-Threatening Illness

9 Do you see a strong-will in your child?

_____

_____

_____

_____

_____

10 Talk with your child about what trips or events he'd enjoy. From that conversation write down a "What's next?" list.

_____

_____

_____

_____

_____

Loneliness—Where are Our Child's Friends?

11 Friendships are a key element in childhood and especially the teen years. Is there a special friend that has been there for your child since the crisis began?

_____

_____

_____

_____

12 If so, talk to your child about what he would like to do the next time he gets together with his friend. List it here.

_____

_____

_____

_____

13 If your child doesn't have a special friend, talk to him about his feelings. Does he ever feel lonely?

_____

_____

_____

_____

14 Is there someone from the clinic with whom he enjoys talking during clinic or hospital visits? If your child is interested, consider how you can help foster new friendships.

_____

_____

_____

_____

15 If he can have a pet, talk to him about getting a pet.

_____

_____

_____

_____

Late-Effect Emotions—Dormant Emotions Erupt After the Crisis

16 Have you noticed warning signs of a possible eruption in your teen?

_____

_____

_____

_____

17 If so, it's time to get serious with God. Pray like his life depends upon it because truthfully it still does. The enemy would love nothing better than for the teen to survive the life-threatening illness only to emerge turning his back on God. Determine a time daily when you will spend time with God praying over your child.

_____

_____

_____

_____

_____

18 In what ways do you see the enemy seeking to kill, steal and destroy (John 10:10)?

_____

_____

_____

_____

19 In countering the enemy's attacks, enlist prayer partners who will commit to praying for you and your teen. List them here.

_____

_____

_____

_____

_____

Caring for the Seriously Ill Child Emotionally—Cheering Him on to Victory

As we learned in the TLC Truth #2: Emotions are a gift from God to be appropriately expressed not suppressed. Children are honest with their emotions. The ways they express or don't express their emotions will vary as much as the individual child.

A child needs time to process what is going on in his life. Open communication appropriate to the child's age is vital. The child may experience feelings of:

- guilt (Was it something I did or didn't do?)
- anger for what happened to him
- envy toward kids who are not sick
- low self-esteem resulting from physical changes
- loss of identity
- loneliness or isolation from friends
- fear of the unknown
- pain from the medicines and procedures
- and fear of death

A parent is the essential piece in the child's emotional peace. We are there for him through the good and the bad, cheering him on to victory. Our number one goal is to be our child's #1 cheerleader. He is going to be up against enough negative opposition from the enemy.

> A parent is the essential piece in the child's emotional peace.

Ways to cheer our child to victory emotionally include open expression of your emotions in front of the child. Modeling that it is okay to cry by crying in front of our child, speaks volumes without ever saying, "It's okay to cry." The child instinctively knows, if mom cries in front of me then it's okay for me to cry in front of her.

If the child is older, respect him by asking for his input on decisions. So much control is taken from the child, especially in the beginning of his journey. Getting his input tells him that he is loved and valued as a person and that his feelings are important.

Another way to cheer our child to victory emotionally is to set him up to succeed in handling his emotions. The unknown is scary to any human, no matter what the age. As adults we try to gather as much information before something happens as possible. Doing the same for our child helps him to know what to expect ahead of time. This helps to relieve anxiety associated with the unknown. It requires that we play detective ahead of time. If we don't have an opportunity to talk in person to the staff before a procedure then we can place a call to the specific area a few days before the procedure. Ask them what to expect from the time we enter the door until we leave. We then have an opportunity at home to explain the procedure to the child. The child has time to process the upcoming procedure. We then have time to allow the child to ask questions. Then, when the actual time comes to have a procedure the child is more confident because he knows what to expect. He feels more in control. The less the anxiety, the more the child is in control of his emotions.

Reflection & Encouragement

"Children's honesty makes it both easier and more heart-wrenching to encounter crises with them. No matter how agonizing the words, accept your child's feelings and your feelings in order to really heal. Denying feelings or holding them in causes a festering wound. As you accept, express, and respond to feelings, you and your child will find healing and wholeness."

—Karen Dockrey

Strength for the Week

Share praises and prayer requests. List them below and pray for these members and their requests throughout the week.

_____

_____

_____

_____

_____

Closing Prayer

Father God, we admit that we can't do this without you. We need your help as we care for our child emotionally. We again praise you that you created emotions to be appropriately expressed and not suppressed. Help us to keep this truth in our mind as our child expresses his emotions. In Jesus' name we pray. Amen.

Week 7 Memory Verse

"Though one may be overpowered, two can defend themselves. A cord of three strands is not quickly broken." (Ecclesiastes 4:12)

Homework

❶ Daily read **TLC Truth** #8: The greatest gift I can give my child is the gift of freedom to be a child to the fullest extent possible.

❷ Read devotional entries 27-29 (beginning on page 147).

❸ Complete Week 8 in preparation for next week's group.

Caring for the Seriously Ill Child Spiritually

Cheering Him on to His Greater Purpose

"'For I know the plans I have for you,' declares the Lord, 'plans to prosper you and not to harm you, plans to give you hope and a future. Then you will call upon me and come and pray to me, and I will listen to you. You will seek me and find me when you seek me with all your heart.'"

—*Jeremiah 29:11-13*

Opening Prayer

Father God, as we focus on caring for our child spiritually, we admit that you must draw him to you. Help us to do our part in leading our child to Jesus. In Jesus' name we pray. Amen.

TLC Truth

#8: The greatest gift I can give my child is the gift of freedom to be a child to the fullest extent possible.

Devotional Questions

God has a Plan and a Purpose for Our Child—Helping Our Child Discover His Purpose

❶ Jean Driscoll is a shining example of how God uses the gifts and talents of a willing vessel. What are your child's interests?

_____

_____

_____

_____

_____

❷ Name some of your child's gifts and talents.

_____

_____

_____

_____

_____

❸ Is there a local event or opportunity to serve in which your child is interested?

_____

_____

_____

_____

_____

❹ Talk to your child about his gifts and talents. Ask him if there is something he would like to do for someone else. Record it and work with your child to make it happen.

_____

_____

_____

_____

_____

Sharing God with Your Child—Do You Know the Great Physician?

❺ Maybe you've gone through this study and have not yet made a decision to trust God with your eternal life. It's not too late. You're still alive. God isn't finished with you yet. He has a plan and a purpose for your life. I encourage you to make your decision today. 2 Corinthians 6:2 tells us, "I tell you, now is the time of God's favor, now is the day of salvation." Salvation is the word used in the Bible when a person realizes he has sinned against God, repents or confesses his sin to God, and commits himself to follow Christ. Don't let another day go without handing your life over to the Divine Healer. Pray from your own heart a prayer similar to this one. Share your decision with the group.

> *Dear Lord, I acknowledge that I have not followed your way. My attempts to save myself have not worked. I ask you to forgive me of all my sin. I believe that you willingly died on the cross for my sins, rose again, and reign as my Savior; thank you that I am now pure in your sight because of what Jesus did on the cross for me. You love me like no other, and desire to come into my life. I accept your gift of salvation. Guide me, Lord, and grant me peace. Thank you. In Jesus' name. Amen.*

If you just prayed this prayer of salvation for the first time, all of heaven is rejoicing! God has saved you from your sin-past, present, and future. He loves you and is with you! He has come into your life, he has given you new life, and he will never leave you (Hebrews 13:5). This is the most crucial decision you can make because not only will your new relationship with Christ influence your life on earth, but it will also assure you of eternal life (1 John 5:12).

---

6 Your child will benefit as you share with him what God is doing and has done in your own life. It will provide building blocks to his faith. What can you share with your child about what God is doing in your life?

Miracles, Faith, Hope, and Healing—"The Other Side of Zero," Part 1

7 Nancy Brown said, "I had prayed to God for Ryan to be healed. Here was my answer. Dr. M was sent by God to help him fix this problem." Do you view your child's medical team as being sent by God to help fix your child's problem?

_____

_____

_____

_____

_____

8 God chooses whatever means to bring healing. He may choose to heal immediately as in the case of Ryan's heart damage or he may choose to heal through medicine he inspires man to create. Sometimes God chooses to postpone healing until heaven. This is a true test of our faith. Have you experienced any of the three ways God chooses to heal? Share your story.

_____

_____

_____

_____

_____

Caring for the Seriously Ill Child Spiritually—Cheering Him On To His Greater Purpose

This is an area where we can only do so much. We can lead the child to Christ but we can't make the child's decision to trust Christ with his earthly and eternal life.

In Matthew 18:14 Jesus tells his disciples "your Father in heaven is not willing that any of these little ones should be lost." Children are special to God. A few verses earlier in verse 10, Jesus tells the disciples, "See that you do not look down on one of these little ones. For I tell you that their angels in heaven always see the face of my Father in heaven." It is reassuring to know that our child has an angel in heaven.

I've known this since 1995. Steve says that Chad's angel has bumps, bruises, scrapes, cuts and a cell phone.

So what's our role in our child's spirituality? Proverbs 22:6 instructs parents to, "Train a child in the way he should go, and when he is old he will not turn from it." Our home is the first place our child is introduced to God's love. You may have just committed your life to Christ during this session and you're not sure exactly what to do as far as the spiritual realm of parenting a child with a life-threatening illness. That's okay. There are wonderful resources and websites offering help in this area. Two great websites are www.family.org and www.troubledwith.com. The first is the official website of Focus on the Family, a non-profit, Christian ministry dedicated to the preservation of the family founded by Dr. James Dobson over twenty-five years ago.

Troubledwith.com is a service of Focus on the Family. It "is a collection of articles, resources and referrals organized by topic around family issues and concerns. The goal is to help families by providing complete coverage of issues including a brief introduction to each topic, an overview of the issue at hand, Q&A with experts and tips for making things better" (www.troubledwith.com).

The greatest way to introduce our child to God is to live the Bible before him—reading the Bible with our child, praying with him and singing children's songs about Jesus. We can fill our home with sights and sounds that bring a spirit of peace with Christian music and media that includes videos and television programs.

The next thing to do is to be available to answer questions from your child when he asks. Again, we don't have to know all of the answers. Let's use these questions as an opportunity to draw our child into the Bible to search for answers. A Bible is the best gift we could give our child.

Memorizing a Bible verse with our child is wonderful, as is playing games using Bible verses (e.g., hangman, crossword puzzles, word searches, etc.). A pastor friend recently underwent a two-hour body scan. He told me the machine made loud noises. To keep his mind off of the noise, he quoted every Bible verse he had ever memorized. The same can be true for our child. When he faces a test where we're not allowed to be in the room, he can find comfort from God's word. Claiming God's promises brings peace to anyone at anytime in anyplace.

So what's our role in our child's spirituality?

The next thing to do is to be available to answer questions from your child when he asks. Again, we don't have to know all of the answers.

Be sure to take our child to church when his health allows it. If his counts don't permit him to be around large crowds, invite his Sunday school teacher to make a home visit with the class lesson. This will be a double blessing. The child will hear about Jesus from someone else, and you will get to enjoy the company of an adult.

Also, join a small group Bible study or continue this group after you finish the curriculum and choose a topical or biblical study on which to focus. Also, look for a church that has a special needs ministry for your child. More churches are realizing the need for such a ministry and many people are responding to the need to serve as leaders in this area.

Finally, we must be faithful in prayer for our child. Enlist prayer partners to continue lifting our child up for spiritual understanding. There is an age where a child knows between right and wrong (sin). That age is different for each child. Only God knows what that age is for our child.

Reflection & Encouragement

"Build a relationship with God that is so reliable you can stake your life on it—because you'll have to.

"We can simply move aside and work along with God as He brings out the childlikeness in our children. We can believe that 'anyone who will not receive the kingdom of God like a little child will never enter it.' (Mark 10:15)'"

—Karen Dockrey

Strength for the Week

Share praises and prayer requests. List them below and pray for these members and their requests throughout the week.

_____

_____

_____

_____

_____

Closing Prayer

Father God, it's hard to comprehend love so strong. It is comforting to know that you want to see my child in heaven more than I want to see my child in heaven someday. Please help me make our home a home made with Jesus' love. Please help me to be patient as my child grows to understand the difference between right and wrong. Help me to answer his questions as honestly as possible and to always turn to the Bible for wisdom and understanding. In Jesus' name I pray. Amen.

Week 8 Memory Verse

"'For I know the plans I have for you,' declares the Lord, 'plans to prosper you and not to harm you, plans to give you hope and a future.'" (Jeremiah 29:11)

Homework

❶ Daily read **TLC Truth #9**: God can provide joy regardless of my circumstances.

❷ Read devotional entries 30-32 (beginning on page 152).

❸ Complete Week 9 in preparation for next week's group.

Caring for the Seriously Ill Child Physically

Cheering Him on to Enjoy Childhood

"The Lord blessed the latter part of Job's life more than the first."

—*Job 42:12*

Opening Prayer

Father God, we praise you that you are a good father. Help us to be mindful that the enemy's goal is to steal our joy. Help us reclaim what rightfully belongs to our children—the joy of childhood. Help us relinquish the identity we have with this crisis and to live out our identity found in you—a child of the king. In Jesus' name. Amen.

TLC Truth

#9: God can provide joy regardless of my circumstances.

Sharing

Share with the group one way that you cheered your child on spiritually this past week. (Did you read the Bible together, sing children's hymns together, watch a Christian video together, work on discovering your child's gifts and talents, etc.?)

Devotional Questions

Everything in Life Can't Be Fun—"The Other Side of Zero",
Part 2

❶ Write about one piece of laughter you have filed in your crisis folder to share with the group at the next session.

_____

_____

_____

_____

_____

❷ Is there one sub-folder that you are allowing too much space in your mind, or allowing it to steal your joy? If so, explain.

_____

_____

_____

_____

_____

Two Wonderful Things Our Children Deserve to Experience—Wishes and Camp

❸ Has your child been granted a wish?

_____

_____

_____

_____

❹ If so, what was your child's wish?

_____

_____

_____

_____

_____

5 If not, consider that your child is well deserving of having a wish granted. Talk to your child about wishes. Write down your child's response.

_____

_____

_____

_____

_____

6 How will you proceed?

_____

_____

_____

_____

7 Has your child gone camping? If so, describe your child's experience.

_____

_____

_____

_____

9 Has your family or your other children gone camping? If so, describe the experience.

_____

_____

_____

_____

Life is a Party—Celebrating the Milestones

❿ Describe celebrations at your home.

_____

_____

_____

_____

_____

⓫ If celebrations are not customary in your home, brainstorm ideas of what you can celebrate and how.

_____

_____

_____

_____

_____

Caring for the Seriously Ill Child Physically—Cheering Him on to Enjoy Childhood

This week we "lighten up and have fun." Job knew what it was to lose everything. In Job 1:8, the Lord describes him as, "blameless and upright, a man who fears God and shuns evil." Yet God allowed the enemy to subject Job to losing his sons, daughters, servants and livestock. He was left with a grumbling wife and three friends that were disciples of doom. In the end, after Job prayed for his friends (there's another lesson), the Lord made him prosperous again and gave him twice as much as he had before.

God had his work cut out for him in getting me to "lighten up." I confess that for the first year and a half I was a stiff, strict mom. One of my jobs was to make sure we played by the doctor's rules. Our house resembled Army barracks more than a home. Whatever the doctor told me to do I did. Steve told me once, "If Dr. K told you to throw Chad off of a building, I think you'd do it without questioning him." For me it was a trust factor. Dr. K trusted me to have enough sense to care for Chad. I didn't want to break that trust. I also trusted him because he had been in this business much longer than I had. It was sort of like what Nancy said, "I had prayed to God for Ryan to be healed. Here was my answer. Dr. M was

> God had his work cut out for him in getting me to "lighten up." I confess that for the first year and a half I was a stiff, strict mom.

sent by God to help him fix this problem." Well, I prayed for God to heal Chad and Dr. K was my answer to help God fix the problem.

God knew I was too reliant on Dr. K. At about the same time Chad came off of the intensive phase of treatment, Steve got a new job out of state. One of the few times I cried was at Chad's last appointment with Dr. K. He did the children's physical for the new school system. Before he sent us on our way he gave us hugs. That's when I lost it.

We moved to Richmond, Virginia with no extended family. Many blessings came from that move. I got to be a stay home mom, again. I met Brenda, my best girl friend and the sister I never had. The best-forced blessing was that I changed my identity.

Before the move to Richmond, I introduced myself as, "I'm Chad's mom. He has leukemia." In the beginning it was therapeutic for me to say it, then it became a habit. My other identities faded. So much of our life initially revolves around the crisis. As the ride begins to settle down, we should return to participating in the things we enjoyed doing before this unwelcome houseguest arrived. We should return to being parents and the children should return to being children. This houseguest should blend in like a piece of furniture.

The move to Richmond was good for me. The move to Baltimore was good for Chad. Education in Richmond became more difficult for Chad with each passing grade. The principals at the schools in Baltimore believe in Chad's abilities. It is so refreshing to attend education meetings and hear praises about what Chad does right in school, not everything he can't do.

This year, I realized, with some help from a friend, I was too over protective in the area of Chad's education. It had turned into a miniature battle of the wills between Chad and "the parents." Chad put his foot down. He expressed his need to be trusted more. He didn't want his homework checked. Thank heavens for the on-line service our school system uses which improves communication between parents, students and teachers. I view Chad's grades at my leisure. This allows him freedom and gives me the assurance I need to still be in the loop.

God doesn't intend for us to live as a slave to this crisis. In referring to money, Jesus told his disciples in Luke 16:13, "'No servant can serve two masters. Either he will hate the one and love the other, or he will be devoted to the one and

Before the move to Richmond, I introduced myself as, "I'm Chad's mom. He has leukemia."

We love the child, not the crisis. Our identity must be in Christ, first and foremost.

despise the other. You cannot serve both God and Money.'" The object we serve doesn't have to be money.

In Mark 12:30 Jesus says that the most important commandment is, "'Love the Lord your God with all your heart and with all your soul and with all your mind and with all your strength.'" The word "all" leaves no room for anything else. We do not love the disease, injury or birth defect, and must be cautious not to give it more room in our heart, soul, mind and strength than it deserves. We love the child, not the crisis. Our identity must be in Christ, first and foremost.

Reflection & Encouragement

"Moving on with life begins by recognizing that crises are interruptions to life, not the end of life. They're a part, not the whole.

"Moving on with life is more than just deciding to grin and bear it. It's grabbing the rays of joy that burst through pinholes in the pain. It's developing techniques and attitudes that enable your child to do his best in spite of the handicap or sadness. It's finding ways to carry the burden or walk around the obstacles. It's confidence that God's power is big enough to manage anything."

—Karen Dockrey

Strength for the Week

Share praises and prayer requests. List them below and pray for these members and their requests throughout the week.

_____

_____

_____

_____

_____

Closing Prayer

Father God, we confess that at times we let this crisis be our identity. Please forgive us for allowing anything to take the place of our identity in you. Help us to recognize ways we need to "lighten up and have fun." Most importantly, help us as we live out the greatest commandment, "Love the Lord your God with all your heart and with all your soul and with all your mind and with all your strength." In Jesus' name we pray. Amen.

Week 9 Memory Verse

> "'Love the Lord your God with all your heart
> and with all your soul and with all your mind
> and with all your strength.'" (Mark 12:30)

Homework

❶ Daily read **TLC Truth #10**: In this world I will have trouble, but I can have peace because Jesus has overcome the world. (from John 16:33)

❷ Read devotional entries 33-39 (beginning on page 158).

❸ Complete Week 10 in preparation for next week's group.

❹ Bring to the next group a scrapbook, photos, drawing, painting, video (check if there's a place to play it) or something that celebrates your child and preserves your child's memory.

Caring for Our Future

Where Do We Go From Here?

"Praise be to the God and Father of our Lord Jesus Christ, the Father of compassion and the God of all comfort, who comforts us in all our troubles, so that we can comfort those in any trouble with the comfort we ourselves have received from God."
—*2 Corinthians 1:3-4*

Opening Prayer

Father God, as we come to the last group session, we thank you for our CarePoint Shepherd and his faithfulness. Thank you also for each member. As parents of seriously ill children, we are assured that our children have not gone through this experience for no reason. Please use this experience to fit in with your plan and purpose for our lives so that ultimately your name will receive praise, honor and glory. In Jesus' name we pray. Amen.

TLC Truth

#10: In this world I will have trouble, but I can have peace because Jesus has overcome the world. (from John 16:33)

Devotional Questions

School and Your Child's Individualized Education Plan—Educating the Educators

❶ Overall, what has been your experience regarding your child's education?

_____
_____
_____
_____

❷ What has been your biggest challenge in working with the school system?

_____
_____
_____
_____
_____

❸ Have you been able to overcome this challenge? If so, how?

_____
_____
_____
_____
_____

Play—When Can I Start Being a Kid Again?

❹ What is your child's favorite form of play?

_____
_____
_____
_____
_____

❺ When was the last time your child got to do his favorite form of play?

_____

6 If your child is not able to engage in this form of play right now, what can you think of to improvise this form of play?

7 Share what area of childhood you have to work at the hardest in order to make childhood happen for your child? Explain your answer.

Survivor's Guilt—The Shadow of Death

8 In what ways has Satan stolen your joy?

9 Have you experienced Survivor's Guilt? If so, how have you handled it?

_____
_____
_____
_____
_____

Pain Management—Being a Strong Advocate

10 In what ways have you been a strong advocate for your child?

_____
_____
_____
_____
_____

11 Can you identify times when you need to be a stronger advocate? If so, what do you think holds you back?

_____
_____
_____
_____
_____

Thy Will Be Done—The Darkest Valley

12 Share your thoughts on the poem "Amazing Child, Amazing Creator vs. Amazing Cancellor"

_____
_____
_____
_____

Death—An Outsider's Observations—We Don't Know How We'll React Until We're In That Position

13 What have you physically comforted your child through? (Survivor's guilt, pain management, the dying process, other.) Share with the group a nugget of hope that you used to cope through this time.

_____

_____

_____

_____

_____

14 Have you experienced the death of a child or someone you loved deeply? If so, describe how that person said goodbye to you. Describe how you said goodbye to that person.

_____

_____

_____

_____

_____

15 Describe the first child you knew who died.

_____

_____

_____

_____

_____

Keeping the Memories Alive—In Life and Death

16 Describe one of your favorite photos of your child, where it was taken, what makes it so special to you, etc.

_____

_____

_____

_____

_____

⓱ Share a story about your child that you want to keep alive.

_____

_____

_____

_____

⓲ Share with the group anything you brought with you (scrapbook, pictures, etc.) to celebrate your child's memory.

_____

_____

_____

_____

_____

We know from our study that sickness, suffering and death are not from God. All good things come from the heavenly Father. God does not waste a bad experience....

Caring for Our Future—Where Do We Go From Here?

As we wrap up our final group session, we turn our attention more closely to the future—our future. Each member of this group has a God given purpose. Our child's illness can be used for good as part of that purpose. We know from our study that sickness, suffering and death are not from God. All good things come from the heavenly Father. God does not waste a bad experience, and his plan is to create beauty from ashes. Romans 8:28 assures us, "And we know that in all things God works for the good of those who love him, who have been called according to his purpose."

Our responsibility is to be listening, praying and sharing. Listen to the Holy Spirit's voice speaking to our hearts. Pray seeking how God wants you to use your gifts, talents and life experiences to accomplish his purpose. Share God's love with those who do not yet know him as personal Savior and Lord of their life.

If our child is still living, we are not finished with the journey. Whatever this journey may bring, God continues to travel with us as long as we continue to invite him to join us. We don't have to be finished with a trip before God can use it for his good. In fact, God values families so much that he allows us to accomplish his purpose for our lives with our family traveling along with us.

For those who have lost a child to death, you must first care for yourself and for your family. I encourage you to take time to grieve. Grief will wait on you. It is a journey that cannot be rushed.

God wants us to mourn. Jesus taught his disciples the importance in mourning. He said, "Blessed are those who mourn, for they will be comforted." He revealed himself as the tender loving comforter in that verse. When we are mourning we need comforting. God doesn't want his children to mourn forever, but he does intend for us to mourn when we experience loss. Jeremiah 31:13 reveals God's plan for his wounded children, "I will turn their mourning into gladness; I will give them comfort and joy instead of sorrow." God alone can do this for us.

There are many wonderful grieving parents' support groups. However, I encourage you to join one that is Bible based. I have seen the evil one pull this trick many times on grieving parents. The enemy offers the hurting parent a bitterness pill. The parent accepts it and swallows it. The bitterness pill is designed to turn your heart away from God. I've seen parents who once were following God begin following a man's philosophy about life and death. Satan's lie is that God took your child. God's truth is that disease, injury or a birth defect took your child's life and that only his love will provide the comfort you need to get through this painful time of your life.

Also, let's not forget about the other members in the family who are hurting too—our spouse and the siblings. We have known too many couples that divorced following the death of their child. Again, unity in God is the key to staying glued together. This is one of the toughest things you and your mate will ever go through. Remember, one of the enemy's greatest threats is the family. He gets no greater joy than to completely destroy a God centered family.

> I have seen the evil one pull this trick many times on grieving parents. The enemy offers the hurting parent a bitterness pill. The parent accepts it and swallows it.

The siblings must be protected against the enemy's destruction plan, too.

The siblings must be protected against the enemy's destruction plan, too. A middle-aged man shared that he felt like "the child who wasn't even there" following his sister's death from an automobile accident.

Role modeling grief for the child is crucial. Demonstrating grief as a natural expression of love for the person who has died shows the sibling that it is okay to cry, to be sad, to be angry, to laugh, to play, and to talk about the child.

No matter which road God takes us down, we drag baggage behind us. This is so true for siblings. They often suffer in silence and mourn in silence. Be assured that they will not always remain silent. Silence does not mean there are no feelings or questions. Talk openly and listen carefully to what they say and to what they do not say.

There may be times when the grief is so great that professional help is in order. If you need to speak with a pastoral or professional Christian counselor, please call the church office listed at the beginning of the workbook for a referral.

Finally, remember to cherish the memories you hold dear in caring for your seriously ill child.

Finally, remember to cherish the memories you hold dear in caring for your seriously ill child. These memories are yet another gift from God. I encourage you to share these memories in some form whether written or verbal with others.

As we come to the close of our time together as a CarePoint small support group, I pray God's continued blessings upon every aspect of your life, especially as a parent caring for a seriously ill child.

Reflection & Encouragement

"I don't know how you would recover from grief without Jesus Christ."

—Dr. Joseph Stowell

"Only eternal confidence brings comfort in human distress."

—Virginia Colclasure

Strength for the Future

Circle up as a group. Lock arms. This represents the bond that has formed over the past ten weeks. It also represents the bond that ties us together as one in the body of Christ.

_____

_____

_____

_____

_____

Closing Prayer

Father God, as our group session comes to a close thank you for friendships that have been formed. Bless each member of our group as we continue caring for our seriously ill child. Continue to equip us to face each challenge with the hope that comes from Jesus Christ, our tender loving comforter. Bind our broken, hemorrhaging hearts with Jesus' healing bandages of love and comfort, and when the burden is too much to bear, remind us that you will carry us, if we will just lift our arms up to you. Finally, help us to cherish the memories we hold dear in caring for our seriously ill child. May they always put a smile on our face even when our heart is breaking. In Jesus' name we pray. Amen.

Week 10 Memory Verse

"I will turn their mourning into gladness; I will give them comfort and joy instead of sorrow." (Jeremiah 31:13)

Homework

Remember TLC Truths:

TLC Truth #1: God cares about my needs.

TLC Truth #2: Emotions are a gift from God to be appropriately expressed not suppressed.

TLC Truth #3: Faith in God can transform me from fearful to fearless.

TLC Truth #4: My body is a temple of the Holy Spirit, designed to bring honor to God.

TLC Truth #5: Families are one of God's greatest treasures on earth to be cherished and protected during the storm.

TLC Truth #6: Humans are God's only creation that worries.

TLC Truth #7: God calls parents to be cheerleaders for their children by encouraging them, comforting them and urging them to live lives worthy of God. (from 1 Thessalonians 2:12)

TLC Truth #8: The greatest gift I can give my child is the gift of freedom to be a child to the fullest extent possible.

TLC Truth #9: God can provide joy regardless of my circumstances.

TLC Truth #10: In this world I will have trouble, but I can have peace because Jesus has overcome the world. (from John 16:33)

Reading Section

1 – Emotions

Straighten Out the Roller Coaster Ride

"For God has said, 'I will never leave you; I will never abandon you.'" (Hebrews 13:5)

In November 1999, our family visited a popular theme park in Florida. Near the end of the day following our souvenir shopping, we headed for a dark inside roller coaster ride, designed to mimic outer space. I climbed on board, fastened my seatbelt and wrapped my arms around gifts intended for the grandparents. This box contained four glass Christmas ornaments.

The unforeseeable twists and turns shocked me. I couldn't anticipate the dips or jerks. Once off of the ride I opened the package to find that two of the four ornaments broke due to the force. However, the other two survived the ride unscathed. How could this be? All four ornaments were subjected to the same twists and turns, yet half of the ornaments crumbled while the other half remained intact.

Often a serious illness is described as riding an emotional roller coaster. Parents of seriously ill children attempt to solve the dilemma by trying to straighten out the roller coaster. This coping mechanism conditions us not to get too high or too low. So instead of riding an emotional roller coaster we find ourselves on a preschool carnival ride going around in a miniature circle at a safe rate of speed.

As good as this plan may sound in theory, and as much as we would love to switch rides, the truth is that we cannot. At this time, we are on an emotional roller coaster ride. We have emotions.

> Often a serious illness is described as riding an emotional roller coaster.

God created us in his likeness and he, too, has emotions. Just like God, we feel things very deeply. His heart breaks for us when our hearts are breaking.

Jesus experienced emotions while he was on earth. He appropriately expressed his emotions. He expressed anger toward the moneychangers at the temple, sadness over the death of his friend, Lazarus, and joy during the wedding feast in Cana. He was in control of his emotions, not controlled by them.

Emotions surface in a variety of ways. My memory fails me when I encounter mega amounts of stress. I misplace items. I am a very organized person. My disorganization is a clear indicator of my state of mind. Following a conversation with a close friend whose son had relapsed with neuroblastoma, I misplaced my contact lens case. I remembered seeing it but could not recall where I had laid it. I found it two weeks later in the trunk of my car.

Steve developed shingles on his face two weeks after Chad's diagnosis. His emotional stress surfaced physically. He stayed at his parents' home next door to us due to Chad's immune-compromised state. He talked to us through the windows. The boys and Steve talked about baseball games over the telephone as they watched them in separate homes. At Chad's one-month bone marrow check, Steve was not allowed to be in the room with us. Our pastor supported me during the procedure. Many times Steve jokingly introduced himself as Job.

> When left to human coping ability, eight words seem to best describe the emotional roller coaster ride: "Get in, sit down, shut up, hold on."

When left to human coping ability, eight words seem to best describe the emotional roller coaster ride: "Get in, sit down, shut up, hold on." However, Psalm 46:10 offers eight alternative coping words when boarding this ride: "Be still, and know that I am God."

Let's scoot over and invite Jesus Christ to ride along in the front seat with us. Then, hand over our most precious ornament, our child, to Jesus. With Christ holding our most treasured gift, we will survive the ride intact.

2 – The Diagnosis

Why?

"We are hard pressed on every side, but not crushed; perplexed, but not in despair." (2 Corinthians 4:8)

Following the pediatric oncologist's pronouncement, his mouth moved, but deafening screams of "no" inside my head silenced his words. An unforeseeable atomic bomb had exploded in my world in the form of a cancer diagnosis for my son.

I mentally reentered Chad's hospital room, to hear the doctor finishing his too-often spoken and too-well memorized "tell the parents" speech. He closed with, "Do you have any questions?" Of course I have questions, but my current state of emotional paralysis allows me only to formulate the two most basic words—two most basic questions—"Why?" and "How?"

He chose to ignore the first question. He could not answer "Why?" These are questions every parent must work through in time: *Why my child? Why me? Why my family? Why?*

The pain that comes with a devastating childhood illness rips the heart open exposing its innermost chambers. During this time of hemorrhaging hurt Satan whispers a lie in our ear, "God did this to your child." God's truth is found in Matthew 5:45. His word tells us "He (God) causes his sun to rise on the evil and the good, and sends rain on the righteous and the unrighteous."

As children of God, we are not immunized against suffering on earth. Suffering has been around since Adam and Eve disobeyed God's command in the Garden of Eden.

We have many different coping skills and emotions when it comes to handling a serious illness. Denial, isolation or loneliness, fear, worry, guilt, anger, bargaining, depression, acceptance, and hope are emotions we may experience.

These emotional stages are normal. It is imperative to realize we may experience these stages many times throughout this journey and not in any particular order.

Some of these emotions may have surfaced before the child's diagnosis. Chad's first symptom, limping, presented three weeks before he was diagnosed. I denied that anything was wrong. Many parents have shared how they explained away their child's initial symptoms. However, finally the symptoms can no longer be ignored.

I also did the bargaining thing. About one week before Chad was diagnosed I played the "Let's Make a Deal" game with God. As Chad lay sleeping beside of me, I quietly sobbed begging God to let me die before Chad. That was my only request. By this time I knew something bad was wrong with him, I just didn't know what.

Anger surfaced about two weeks following diagnosis. I didn't aim my anger at God (in my thinking, that would have

> The pain that comes with a devastating childhood illness rips the heart open exposing its innermost chambers.

been disrespectful). I displaced all of my anger onto my mother-in-law. Not three days passed until Chad developed a fever requiring hospitalization. That was when my emotional roller coaster car derailed. The results of the initial bone marrow test revealed a high risk factor. This meant not three chemotherapies but eight during the cycle to include bi-weekly hospitalizations. We were in an entirely new arena. The percentages for survival plunged.

I heard God speaking to me as Dr. K finished another speech, "Rita, I'm still in control here. Your attitude can make this or break this. It's your choice."

As soon as I got home that night I called my mother-in-law. She entered our bedroom to hear me hysterically crying for her forgiveness.

I was angry with God for allowing this to happen to Chad. I bought into Satan's lie that God allowed this to happen to Chad. I learned to talk to God about my anger.

Satan's goal is to drive a barrier of bitterness between God and us. He plants the false lie that we are better off without God.

Choose to continue on with God. It is healthy to release resentment we may be harboring against God. The best way to break down any barrier is to keep the lines of communication open. We communicate with God by praying or talking to him. He communicates with us when we read his word and the Holy Spirit speaks to our quieted soul. Isaiah 26:2 promises, "You (God) will keep in perfect peace him whose mind is steadfast, because he trusts in you."

Begin by telling God exactly how you feel. Unload every emotion you're feeling. He can handle our doubt, anger, fear, worry, grief, confusion, and questions. In Job 7:11, Jobs says, "Therefore I will not keep silent; I will speak out in the anguish of my spirit, I will complain in the bitterness of my soul." God lovingly listened to Job and he lovingly listens to us.

David and Job spent much time talking straight up to God about their feelings. God never intended for us to walk through valleys of fear, insecurity and uncertainty alone. He gives us strength if we ask him for it.

> It is healthy to release resentment we may be harboring against God.

3 – The Blame Game

How?

> *"As he went along, he saw a man blind from birth. His disciples asked him, 'Rabbi, who sinned, this man or his parents, that he was born blind?' 'Neither this man nor his parents sinned,' said Jesus, 'but this happened so that the work of God might be displayed in his life.'"* (John 9:1-3)

A platoon of white coats march in and out of our child's hospital room like it has a revolving door. They seem to ask the same questions. They want to know our family's life details before diagnosis. They ask questions about previous family generations. They ask about the pregnancy. Sometimes they ask questions that only God can answer.

The most important thought to keep in mind during this "interrogation process" is that birth defects and diseases still puzzle the medical community. The truth is that doctors do not have the answers to what causes some diseases and birth defects. Even if they do know the cause of the illness they still do not know how to prevent it. They are learning, too. They ask questions searching for missing puzzle pieces to not only cure diseases and birth defects but to prevent them.

Jesus' disciples looked to place blame for the blind man's condition. Jesus told them the truth. "'Neither this man nor his parents sinned,' said Jesus, 'but this happened so that the work of God might be displayed in his life.'" (John 9:3)

Blame is a waste of time that can eat us alive. Placing blame is another avenue to displace our anger. Instead of properly dealing with our anger we step into a cycle similar to a dog chasing its tail. Nothing productive is ever accomplished. Instead let's heed Jesus' word to the disciples in John 9:13: Give God praise when he works for good in our children's lives. Even if nothing spectacular appears to be happening still give praise to God for waking us up each morning. Choosing to magnify God's work in our circumstances reinforces our dependence upon him.

"Don't try to figure out how Chad got cancer. You'll never be able to figure it out. You'll drive yourselves crazy," the medical staff told us.

Guard yourself against being drawn into Satan's lie called the blame game. His goal is to convince us we did or did not do something that caused our child's disease or birth defect. The truth is that as loving parents there is no way we would

Jesus' disciples looked to place blame for the blind man's condition. Jesus told them the truth.

ever allow this to happen to our children. As Chad appropriately says, "It's just life."

Another version of the blame game is that we blame ourselves or our doctors for the delay in our child's diagnosis. For three weeks two different doctors insisted Chad's illness was a virus. One doctor laughed when Steve told him that we were thinking the worst. The doctor asked, "What do you think is wrong with Chad?" Steve replied, "I think it is either MS or leukemia." The doctor sneered, "It's not leukemia. We've checked him for that!" That doctor never paid us a social visit following diagnosis.

My choice was to harbor bitterness and blame the doctors or to praise God for his provision of a doctor who listened to us with a mother's heart. A female pediatrician had returned from maternity leave. She believed me when I told her that there was something bad wrong with him and that I just didn't know what it was.

When Chad was diagnosed, 80% of his bone marrow was cancer. Because of his high risk factor (fast cancer) he was dying before our eyes. Again, praise God the disease was finally diagnosed and Chad is still alive.

Let's not waste one sweet second of today living bitterly in the past. Let's choose to say as the psalmist did in Psalm 118:24: "This is the day the Lord has made; let us rejoice and be glad in it."

> Another lie of Satan's is that God did this to our child as a punishment for a past sin we committed.

Another lie of Satan's is that God did this to our child as a punishment for a past sin we committed. Jesus does not condemn. The Holy Spirit convicts us of our sin. God's word tells us in Romans 3:23 "for all have sinned and fall short of the glory of God." This is why Jesus came to earth. Verse 25 tells us, "God presented him (Jesus) as a sacrifice of atonement, through faith in his blood."

Satan tries to snare spouses into placing blame on their mate. At one of the most difficult times in a marriage, the last thing the marriage needs is a crippling game of blame. More will be said on marriage later in the workbook. For now a word to the wise is, don't place blame on your mate, and if you are already doing it, stop immediately.

4 – Shattered Dreams

Grieving the Child Who Will Not Exist

> *"So David and his men wept aloud until they had no strength left to weep." (1 Samuel 30:4)*

Larkspur Summerville said, "If Jesus came down right now and sat on the end of my bed, He'd see me crying again, and He'd offer His sleeve, so I might lay my face on His forearm and let my tears soak into the white of His garment. It would be a river of tears. And the sleeve would never become heavy and sopping because no matter how many I cried, He could dry them with plenty of soft, dry comfort."

Although Larkspur is a fictional character in the novel *Women's Intuition* written by Lisa Samson, she eloquently expresses how it is to grieve and to be comforted by Jesus, our tender, loving comforter.

The truth is that when we become parents of seriously ill children we must go through a grieving process of sorts. Although our child is alive, we must grieve for the child who will not be as we had thought he or she would be in our minds.

No matter the circumstance, we must grieve for the child we will not have. If the child has a birth defect, we begin grieving when the defect is discovered by the doctor, either prior to or after the birth of the baby. If the child is diagnosed with a life-threatening illness we begin grieving at diagnosis. If the child is injured in a life-altering accident we begin grieving upon learning of the child's accident.

This is a normal part of the process of coming to terms with the disease, defect or accident. We must grieve and release the part of our child that no longer exists, in order to move forward and effectively deal with the child's life now.

We must grieve and release the part of our child that no longer exists, in order to move forward and effectively deal with the child's life now.

One mother believes the parents who grieve the most are those who have a child with a birth defect. She explained that at least the parents of a child diagnosed with a disease or in an accident did get to experience a child living a "normal" life for a period of time.

Others would argue the opposite. They say it is better to never experience a normal childhood than to have it stolen.

Either viewpoint brings us to the reality that as parents of a seriously ill child we MUST grieve for the child who will no longer exist. Just like grief associated with a death, this grieving process will wait for us until we address it.

My safe place to grieve was in the shower each morning as Chad slept in the hospital bed. I found it therapeutic to cleanse my mind and heart. Romans 8:26 assures us, "the Spirit helps us in our weakness. We do not know what we ought to pray for, but the Spirit himself intercedes for us with groans that words cannot express." I know the Holy Spirit interceded on my behalf during those mornings when I couldn't even pray. All I could do was cry and shake. By the end of my therapy session/shower God filled my heart with thanksgiving. I walked out into the hospital room blessed to enjoy another day with my child who was surviving cancer.

Also, we revisit the grieving process throughout our child's life. Living life will cause us to revisit and re-grieve. As Chad grows I find myself grieving for areas of his life that are more difficult than his sister or brother's, like education and socialization. Again, God is faithful. I continue to ask him for strength and he is faithful to give me strength.

> Satan also invites us to play the game of resentment and envy. These are friendship barriers between God and us.

Satan also invites us to play the game of resentment and envy. These are friendship barriers between God and us. Somewhere along this journey, we may find ourselves looking at parents of healthy children with feelings of resentment or envy. Although we never want another parent to go through what we are, we still may think, "You don't have a clue how fortunate you are to not be walking in my shoes. Do you know how lucky you are?" You are happy for other parents who have healthy children. As my friend, Brenda, mother of Holly, a special daughter with a "special heart," said, "Oh, yeah, I'm so happy I'm gritting my teeth."

Instead of dwelling on what our children will miss in life, choose to look forward to what our children will do—find a cure for cancer, find a prevention for a birth defect, or invent medical equipment to aid in the enhancement of life. God does not see diseases or disabilities; he only sees vessels available to be used by the Master. Wallpapering our minds with the truth from Jeremiah 29:11, "'For I know the plans I have for you,' declares the Lord, 'plans to prosper you and not to harm you, plans to give you hope and a future'" gives us assurance that he is in control and has a great plan.

5 – If

Today Our Child is Living with (fill in your child's illness, injury or birth defect)

> *"'Therefore do not worry about tomorrow, for tomorrow will worry about itself. Each day has enough trouble of its own.'" (Matthew 6:34)*

"If" deals with regrets of the past (If only...) and worries of the future (What if...?). There is no room for the word "if" in the word "today."

We recall hurts from the past following a tragic event. These memories bring regrets and sadness. We all have regrets from the past: an ill-spoken word, too harsh of a punishment, too high expectations, or an unfulfilled promise to our child.

Regrets of the past are just that, in the past. Yesterday's door does not allow reentrance to correct our mistakes. Yesterday's "should have" and "could have" can be turned into today's "will" and "can."

Satan whispers lies that we can't change the way we do things or the way we deal with people. This lie keeps us in bondage from freedom found in Christ.

God's truth is that we can learn from our mistakes of yesterday vowing with God's help not to repeat those mistakes. Praise God we do not have to remain in the past. God is a God of no regrets. I love the way Marlene Bagnull beautifully explains the past, "While some opportunities may be gone forever, God does not leave me in the land of regrets. He redeems the time I've lost and gives me another chance." She uses the scripture reference Proverbs 28:13: "He who conceals his sins does not prosper, but whoever confesses and renounces them finds mercy."

After diagnosis I worried about the future. At first mentally and then audibly, I said to myself, "Stop. Stop. Stop. Don't borrow trouble from tomorrow we have enough trouble today." (My paraphrased version of Matthew 6:34) Satan lures us to play the "What If" mind game. It's another of Satan's lies that can drive us crazy if we play it to the end. Our minds' ability is to go from A to ZZ in record-breaking speed. If Chad experienced one symptom my mind traveled to the land of death and dying.

Over time we realize that not all die from our child's illness. Many survive and thrive. Every day our child wakes is another day he is living with and surviving the illness.

Each day is a new day. Each day begins as a clean slate. Choose this day to live in the present; no ifs, ands, or buts.

6 – Fear of Death

Facing our Greatest Fear

"Even though I walk through the valley of the shadow of death, I will fear no evil, for you are with me" (Psalm 23:4)

Regrets of the past are just that, in the past. Yesterday's door does not allow reentrance to correct our mistakes.

Tragedy forces parents to face our ultimate fear—fear of our own death. This requires that we admit we are mortal, too.

Death is the last thing we want to think about following our child's diagnosis. However, we must come to terms with our own death before we can help our child come to terms with his death. Without facing our own death we can't be reassuring when the subject comes up from our child. This subject will come up because Ecclesiastes 3:11 tells us "He (God) has also set eternity in the hearts of men."

Our earthly life is the dress rehearsal for eternity. Our physical death begins our eternal spiritual life. The question is which life? God's word describes our eternal life two ways; either in the presence of Jesus Christ or in darkness eternally removed from him.

Asking Christ to be our personal Savior is the first, and most important, step on our journey of caring for our seriously ill child. He meets us where we are, and leads us where we need to go.

Recall the imagery of handing our most treasured ornament, our child, over to Jesus while on this emotional roller coaster ride. As parents, we are treasured in Christ's eyes as much as our child.

He died on the cross for every human's sin. He donated his healing blood and sinless life on the cross so that everyone who believes in his name and accepts his free gift for our sins will have eternal life in the presence of Jesus Christ, our tender loving Comforter. Three days later God revived Jesus' dead body and resurrected him (took his body back into heaven). He is alive now. Jesus conquered our greatest fear—death. His only requirement is that we hand over our life to him. We, too, must willingly allow him to hold us for the rest of our physical life.

Carmen Leal, author of *The Twenty-Third Psalm for Caregivers*, has created a beautiful website (www.thetwentythird psalm.com/movie). Visit the site and be blessed.

> We must come to terms with our own death before we can help our child come to terms with his death.

7 – Fear and Faith

From Fearful to Fearless

"So do not fear, for I am with you; do not be dismayed, for I am your God. I will strengthen you and help you; I will uphold you with my righteous right hand." (Isaiah 41:10)

Faith

What is faith?
Is it something you can feel or see?
I think not...
It is something you must believe...

When the future is not clear,
And the present is not bright,
Do not have fear,
But spark your world with the Light,

As you may be afraid,
To open a new door,
Don't worry,
For God will hold up your world...

So do not fret,
Or have dread,
But trust God,
For he is the one who gives you faith.

—Katie Gray

Our daughter expresses her thoughts through poetry. She wrote this for a school assignment while Chad was going through treatments. It gives us a glimpse into her feelings and reveals in whom she places her trust.

Initially, we may feel uncomfortable and incapable of caring for our child. We all experience these feelings. The truth is that God doesn't call the qualified. God qualifies the called. At the onset we may not feel qualified to do this job, but remembering that God is our helper offers us reassurance. All we need to do is to ask him for help. Prayer is a confidence builder. Proverbs 1:7 says, "The fear of the Lord is the beginning of knowledge." The fear of the Lord involves acknowledging God's power and sovereignty.

The phrase "do not be afraid" is in the Bible more times than any other phrase. He knows that without him we are cowards. Fear of the Lord is the only fear he wants us to possess.

God's chosen leaders made excuses. In Judges 6 and 7, before there was any evidence that Gideon was a fearless military leader the angel of the Lord said to Gideon, "The Lord is with you, mighty warrior"(Judges 6:12). Gideon certainly did not feel like a warrior. He reminded the Lord in verse 15, "'But Lord,' Gideon asked, 'how can I save Israel? My clan is the weakest in Manasseh, and I am the least in my family.'" But the Lord looked right past the excuse and assured Gideon

> The truth is that God doesn't call the qualified. God qualifies the called.

what he was going to do for him and what Gideon was going to do. "The Lord answered, 'I will be with you, and you will strike down all the Midianites together.'" Still, verse 27 tells us that he was afraid of his family. He did what the Lord instructed him to do at night instead of day. But when the Spirit of the Lord came upon Gideon, he went from being fearful to being fearless. In Judges 7:17 he told his army, "Watch me. Follow my lead. When I get to the edge of the camp, do exactly as I do." No fear, just a mighty warrior.

Faith requires moving past the excuses. At some point in our care giving role, we must choose to trust God—asking him to help us not be afraid of the journey that lies before us but instead inviting him to help us in this role. We can make excuses of why we don't feel adequate to care for our child. Truthfully, without God's help, we are inadequate for this task. However, as a child of God, he qualifies us to do more than we can think or imagine because we are doing it with his power at work within us (Ephesians 3:20-21). He can change us from a fearful coward to a "fearless caregiver."

> *Truthfully, without God's help, we are inadequate for this task.*

8 – Prayer

The Most Powerful Medicine

"Pray without ceasing...." (1 Thessalonians 5:17)

From day one of diagnosis folks were praying for us. Jerry, our Sunday school teacher and a licensed psychiatrist, was outside of the room when Dr. K announced Chad's diagnosis. He came in after Dr. K left, and we shared our news with him. He was on his way to Wednesday evening prayer service, so he prayed for us then left on a mission. He started the prayer chain at our home church.

Also, that afternoon Steve contacted other pastors to begin prayer chains. One pastor stepped out of his church service to take Steve's call, then went back into the service and called the congregation to the altar to pray for us.

How comforting it is to be wrapped in prayer! Cards came from out of state folks telling us they were praying because someone requested prayer for us. There's great comfort knowing God's family is petitioning the throne of God on behalf of our child.

> *How comforting it is to be wrapped in prayer!*

My great-grandmother followed the instructions in James 5:14-16, "Is any one of you sick? He should call the elders of the church to pray over him and anoint him with oil in the name of the Lord. And the prayer offered in faith will make the sick person well; the Lord will raise him up. If he has sinned, he will be forgiven. Therefore confess your sins to each other and pray for each other so that you may be healed. The prayer of a righteous man is powerful and effective." Elders of her church anointed a white handkerchief with oil and prayed for Chad. She mailed it to me. The handkerchief traveled with us to all doctor appointments and hospital treatments.

In Matthew 18:19 Jesus instructed his disciples on prayer: "Again, I tell you that if two of you on earth agree about anything you ask for, it will be done for you by my Father in heaven. For where two or three come together in my name, there am I with them." Jesus Christ is our best advocate.

We must pray not only for our child, but also for our child's doctors. God can use them, the medicine, and whatsoever he chooses to work on behalf of our child.

Jesus Christ is our best advocate.

9 – God's Promises in the Bible

At the Least Comfort/At the Best Healing

"Let the word of Christ dwell in you richly as you teach and admonish one another with all wisdom, and as you sing psalms, hymns and spiritual songs with gratitude in your hearts to God." (Colossians 3:16)

The hand-written note said:

Rita,

Here are a few of the scriptures I keep in my Bible and read daily. There are many more on the tape. (A cassette tape was enclosed in the envelope.)

Psalm 103:3   Matthew 4:23
Psalm 107:20   Matthew 9:20-22
Isaiah 53:5   Luke 6:19
Jeremiah 30:17   James 5:14-15
Proverbs 4:20-22   Hebrews 13:8
Proverbs 3:8   2 Corinthians 5:7
1 Peter 2:24   Hebrews 11:6
Matthew 9:35

I hope they are as much a comfort to you as they are to me…Keep us in your prayers & we'll do the same. Take care—

Love,

P & boys

Praying is our way of talking to God. Reading and meditating on God's word is God's way of talking to us. Meditating on God's word changes our focus from our worries to God's promises to us. God's words offer comfort and healing to our soul.

Paul said in 2 Corinthians 1:3-5, "Praise be to the God and Father of our Lord Jesus Christ, the Father of compassion and the God of all comfort, who comforts us in all our troubles, so that we can comfort those in any trouble with the comfort we ourselves have received from God. For just as the sufferings of Christ flow over into our lives, so also through Christ our comfort overflows."

Psalm 119:105 reassures us that, "Your word is a lamp to my feet and a light for my path."

10 – Loneliness

Where is God?

> *"Do not be afraid or discouraged because of this vast army. For the battle is not yours, but God's."*
> *(2 Chronicles 20:15)*

"You do realize that God is carrying you right now?" our pastor said to me as I slumped in the chair beside Chad's bed. I couldn't hide my exhaustion. He went on to explain that when we get so tired and don't feel like we can go on, that is when Jesus picks us up in his loving arms and carries us, giving us time to rest. Without me realizing it, Jesus was carrying me.

A plane trip gave another perspective on the same promise. Dark rain clouds blanketed the airport. The plane rose above the clouds revealing the bright sunshine. The sun was shining over the airport, too. We just couldn't see it for the storm clouds. The Son is always there even when we don't feel his presence. That's the difference between faith and feelings.

Satan wants us to operate on feelings. He knows we will not always feel close to God. Sometimes when a life storm comes we may experience depression. In Julia Scott's CarePoint workbook entitled Coveting the Sky: Finding Your Wings in Depression's Storm, she states, "It is imperative that you seek

Satan wants us to operate on feelings. He knows we will not always feel close to God.

the help of a doctor so that you can determine if you have physical problems that are either causing or contributing to your depression. Just as all snowflakes are intricately different, so are each person's brain, health, and personal experiences; thus, there is no one sure healing path for all—we travel according to the individualized healing our particular illness requires! So, first, determine if your illness stems from internal factors (brain chemistry, hormones, other sickness in the body) or external factors (life experiences, post-partum, and environment) or both!"

I did not experience depression during Chad's cancer. However, I did when Steve was in a head-on automobile accident, had fusion surgery on his neck and then developed a deep vein thrombosis (DVT). I went into a state of deep depression. I sought the help of my family doctor. Medication and prayers for me by family and friends brought me through one of the roughest periods of my life. I believe I experienced depression because it was the first time that I had to go through a traumatic life experience without my best friend and mate. During our other life experiences, we went through them together as a team.

Faith believes the Son is there even when we can't see him. David, described as a man after God's own heart, questions God throughout Psalms concerning his closeness. In Psalm 22:11 David begs God, "Do not be far from me, for trouble is near and there is no one to help." David experienced loneliness and depression.

Faith believes the Son is there even when we can't see him.

Jesus experienced loneliness while on earth. In John 16:32 he told his disciples, "But a time is coming and has come, when you will be scattered, each to his own home. You will leave me all alone. Yet I am not alone, for my Father is with me.

However, a time came when even God was not with his son. The loneliest time in the history of man was when God turned his back on his only son, Jesus Christ, because he was bearing the sin of the world while on the cross. Mark 15:34 says, "And at the ninth hour Jesus cried out in a loud voice, 'Eloi, Eloi, lama sabacthani?'—which means, 'My God, my God, why have you forsaken me?'"

We, who have accepted his gift of forgiveness of our sins, will never be alone because the Holy Spirit lives in our hearts. We can cry out to him during these lonely, depressing storms of life.

11 – Rest

A Gift from God

> *"By the seventh day God had finished the work he had been doing; so on the seventh day he rested from all his work. And God blessed the seventh day and made it holy, because on it he rested from all the work of creating that he had done."* (Genesis 2:2-3)

It's okay to reshuffle or delete items off of our "To Do" list or our "Dream List." With our new role we now have new priorities. God wants us to hand over our calendar to him. Daily ask God to order our day allowing him to accomplish through us his most important priorities for us.

Then, let go of the rest. Rest in him. Physical, emotional and spiritual rest is necessary for this journey. Napping while our child naps is refreshing. Letting the answering machine do the job it was designed for is healthy.

Follow God's lead. Observe the Sabbath and keep it holy. It's God prescription for rest. He did it. If it was good for him then it's good for us.

Jump into Jesus' loving arms saying to him, "Hold Me. I'm not strong enough to walk. I need for you to carry me through this valley." David describes the Lord as our shepherd in Psalm 23 verse 2 who "makes me lie down in green pastures, he leads me beside quiet waters, he restores my soul." Allow him to do the same for you.

Also, we must rest our minds. Avoid borrowing trouble from the future. Instead focus on the present—the truth. The truth is that our child is being treated. When despairing thoughts creep into our minds, turn to God asking him to quiet our minds and to direct our thoughts to focus on the present and the blessings we have close at hand—our child.

> Physical, emotional and spiritual rest is necessary for this journey.

12 – Nutrition and Exercise

Loving Ourselves

> *"Do you not know that your body is a temple of the Holy Spirit, who is in you, whom you have received from God? You are not your own; you were bought at a price. Therefore honor God with your body."* (1 Corinthians 6:19-20)

Our eating habits are an easy way to live out our emotions while going through this journey. Too often we eat because of our emotional state, not because our stomachs are growling. My friend Christine, whose eighteen-month-old son, Daniel, died from a brain tumor, expressed so well what our physical appearance is, "It is a shield. It's an outward expression to others about how you are doing emotionally."

I dealt with stress through my mouth. It's really easy to do. The hospital encouraged the parents to check on the menu what we thought the kids might eat. We could also write in special requests that weren't on the menu. A tray full of food would come into the room. Chad would look at it and shake his head no. I would go to work on it, cramming down every morsel before the tray was taken away. I always managed not to waste a crumb.

I dealt with stress through my mouth. It's really easy to do.

I continued to put on weight. By the end of Chad's hospital treatment phase of his protocol I weighed as much as when I was nine months pregnant.

I determined that it was time to take control of my weight. I began planning my meals and drinking water. I didn't eat off of Chad's tray. I went to the cafeteria before his breakfast tray came. I was doing all of the right things but the pounds weren't budging.

It is of the utmost importance to continue getting regular check-ups. I take medication for a hypoactive thyroid. Every six months I have blood work to monitor my thyroid level.

Finally, I decided to go to the doctor. My thyroid had lost some more function and the medicine needed to be increased. The medication level went up and the weight went down by 30 pounds.

Walking is the one exercise that nearly all of us can do. We may only be able to take a step or two starting out, but it is a start.

Taking care of our body is mandatory. There's not another one like us and there is no one else who can love and care for our child the way we can. Our children need us. We want to live to see them grow up.

Taking care of our body is mandatory.

13 – Real Friends / Support Groups

It's Okay to Cry

> *"Though one may be overpowered, two can defend themselves. A cord of three strands is not quickly broken."*
> (*Ecclesiastes 4:12*)

Donna, Penny and I were a trio in the pediatric oncology unit. Our three boys were diagnosed fairly close in time. They were buds in the hospital.

Together, we celebrated milestones and cried over set-backs. Donna's family celebrated Chad's 6th birthday with us. A family photo shows Donna with a glow on her face. They had everything to be smiling about. Her son had been given a clean bill of health in January at a world-renowned children's hospital in Memphis, Tennessee following a bone marrow transplant. He had his double Hickman catheter removed. In another photo our boys looked like brothers—blond hair, same height, both so healthy and smiling as they hugged each other. That was February.

Unsuccessful telephone calls left me with a gut feeling that something was wrong. Upon making contact with Donna, my feeling was validated. They had not been home because her son had relapsed. They had been in Memphis.

"Oh, Donna, I am so sorry" was all that I could strain through my wobbly voice as I sobbed. Donna was crying, too. She said, "Rita, I'm scared to death he is going to die."

No, this is not what I want to hear, I thought as she spoke those words. How can she utter such words? Please don't say that, I thought in denial and shock.

> Donna had already gone to a place I didn't want to ever go.

Donna had already gone to a place I didn't want to ever go. I listened and cried as she shared her heart, her fears, and her plans for the future.

The next phone call I made to Donna was the last time her son was in the hospital. Dr. K had told them to take him home to die. There was nothing else they could do for him. The phone rang to his room and Penny answered. Penny was sitting with him while Donna went home to get his room ready. Once again three friends laughed and cried together.

The phone rang on a Sunday morning in May. Penny said, "Rita." The tears in my eyes and the lump in my throat made it difficult to even ask questions. The night of visitation Penny and I arrived at the funeral home at the same time. We walked through the receiving line together. Hugs, tears, and love surrounded this trio of mothers who bonded in friendship.

Later that year, Donna took a position at school as an aide to Penny's son. Once again, I received a phone call, this time from Donna. Penny's son had relapsed. Donna shared how she was reliving all that she went through with her son.

And again, a phone call, this time from Donna, told me that Penny's son had gone to be with God. Sorrow flooded my soul again. My heart broke all over again.

That was five years and two moves ago. I have been blessed to meet a new group of cancer moms at Mountain Christian Church. There's Christine, Connie, Kathy, Nancy, and Virginia. These ladies and Brenda, my special sister-in-Christ in Richmond, are all contributors to this workbook. Brenda is the mom of Holly, a very special young lady with a special heart. Our experiences have common threads woven through them. Brenda's name should be listed on the by-line.

Oh yes, Kathy called yesterday, her seven-year-old son was declared in remission last week. The doctor told her that when he first saw him that he considered him incurable. We both yelled, "Praise the Lord! Praise God!" in unison over the phone. She stopped by so we could give each other a real hug. She jumped out of the van and we hugged in the driveway. Tears of joy and relief gushed from Kathy. I never tire of hugging a friend and letting her cry tears of relief and joy on my shoulder.

This is what this group is all about—friendships and connecting with fellow sojourners, celebrating in the great times and crying together in the bad times. I praise God that he dreams bigger than I dream. I only envisioned writing a book of emotional devotionals, not of being part of a small support group ministry where parents are encouraged to bond, share, love and support others in similar situations.

This is what this group is all about—friendships and connecting with fellow sojourners, celebrating in the great times and crying together in the bad times.

14 – Attitude of Gratitude

"Someone's not Happy but We are."

> *"A cheerful heart is good medicine, but a crushed spirit dries up the bones." (Proverbs 17:22)*

In the faint distance at the opposite end of the hallway we heard the screams of a very unhappy pediatric patient. We could not determine the age but from the sound of the cry one thing was obvious—this small patient was not happy.

The nurse was changing Chad's bed linens. With a truthful heart Chad announced, "Someone's not happy but we are." I had to smile with joy and give him a great big hug. There he sat with a bald head from chemotherapy, pale skin from lack of an immune system and confined to four small walls for four days. His nurse said, "Oh, Chad, I just have to give your little bald head a kiss because I don't hear my patients say that."

The apostle Paul wrote in Philippians 4:11 that he had "learned to be content whatever the circumstances." Tom Randall, the Chaplain for the Senior PGA Tournament explains it this way, "Grateful people are happy people." As parents of seriously ill children, we often have reminders around us that our child could be even worse off. We have everything to be thankful for.

It's good for us to express our gratitude to God and to those around us. In Luke 17:11-19, ten men with leprosy called out to Jesus in a loud voice, "'Jesus, Master, have pity on us!'" He gave them instruction to go show themselves to the priests. "'And as they went, they were cleansed.'" Verses 15-19 say, "One of them, when he saw he was healed, came back, praising God in a loud voice. He threw himself at Jesus' feet and thanked him—and he was a Samaritan. Jesus asked, 'Were not all ten cleansed? Where are the other nine? Was no one found to return and give praise to God except this foreigner?' Then he said to him, 'Rise and go; your faith has made you well.'"

Jesus healed ten but only one came back to give gratitude. Praise and thanksgiving please God. Take every opportunity to brag on God and all of his glorious blessings. Our culture expects us to be griping and complaining.

We must be mindful that through our attitude is our spiritual thermometer. Unexpressed gratitude can be interpreted as ingratitude. We can lose the loyalty of people because of ingratitude. Ingratitude can even be interpreted as arrogance, then decadence, next narcissism sets in, then an attitude of entitlement; next higher expectations take hold, and finally disappointment, anger and ingratitude to the point that all perspective is gone.

American culture teaches us to be particular. However, during this journey we are going to encounter so many wonderful, giving, loving people that are going to do errands for us, make food for us, take our other children to practices for us, tutor our children, clean our home, do our laundry, etc. that we need to be mindful to have the attitude of gratitude. Although we may be exhausted, let's not forget to say thank you, send a note card of thanks, hug them and verbally express just how much they mean to us. The truth is that we cannot be everything to everybody on this journey and we must be keenly aware of expressing our appreciation to these wonderful people with servant's hearts.

> Jesus healed ten but only one came back to give gratitude. Praise and thanksgiving please God.

15 – Perseverance / Admit Our Weaknesses

Strength for the Day / Ask for Help

> *"Three times I pleaded with the Lord to take it away from me.*
> *But he said to me, 'My grace is sufficient for you, for my*
> *power is made perfect in weakness.' Therefore I will boast all*
> *the more gladly about my weaknesses, so that Christ's power*
> *may rest on me. That is why, for Christ's sake, I delight in*
> *weaknesses, in insults, in hardships, in persecutions, in diffi-*
> *culties. For when I am weak, then I am strong."*
> *(2 Corinthians 12:8-10)*

The apostle Paul shares his pleas to God with the Corinthian church. Three times he asked God to remove his "thorn." God's reply to Paul was for him to continue trusting. Depending on God in our weakness gives us reason to brag on God. James 4:6 says, "God opposes the proud but gives grace to the humble."

Up until Chad's diagnosis I was a one-man show. People offered help when Chad had his accident. I don't remember accepting one offer though.

Then the bomb dropped. The Holy Spirit prodded me to accept help from day one. In my own strength I wanted to handle it all. I had to release my desire to handle the practical physical aspects without any help from friends and relatives. Sometimes God comes on the scene himself to help in a situation and other times God sends people to the scene to help us. This is God's gift to us. He sends people who want to extend hugs, comfort and love.

Believing we can handle everything on our own strength is a lie from Satan. God did not make people to be individual islands. He made man for fellowship and community. We are better together.

We received cards and letters from folks we had never met as well as practical help from people we'd never met. One lady from church made Katie's cheerleading outfit. Aunt Amy purchased the material for the outfit. Our Sunday school department left boxes of low sodium food on our doorstep and had pizza delivered pre-paid following hospital stays. Homemade bread was delivered. Church friends delivered daily meals for a month. A retired teacher offered homework help. The parents of the children's friends took Katie and Ryan on weekend field trips. Our Sunday school class and our co-workers delivered envelopes of cash. Our mothers took over the duties I was unable to do from a hospital room.

> Sometimes God comes on the scene himself to help in a situation and other times God sends people to the scene to help us.

They did laundry, cooked meals and loved and cared for the children. Girl friends from our Sunday school class brought lunch to me. We ate together while a nurse sat with Chad. One gentleman made hospital visits while we were doing weekly treatments. For eight months he stopped in to visit on his way to work.

Countless other ways, real life ways, loving people reached out to us. We were overwhelmed by everyone's love and generosity. "Thank you" seems so inadequate to say. However, they weren't doing it for praise. They were doing it because of their love for us and, more importantly, their love for Christ. They were the hands of Christ.

Some things only God can do for us—give us strength and hope. I remember sharing my concerns with our family pastor, Ira, the night Chad was diagnosed. I was concerned about my ability to be in the room with Chad while they performed the bone marrow aspiration the next morning. Ira's words still burn in my mind; "God will give you the strength to cross the bridge when you are taking the first step to go across the bridge, not one mile from the bridge."

God's mercies are new each day. In our weaknesses we are the strongest. By asking for help God renews our strength daily.

> Some things only God can do for us—give us strength and hope.

16 – The Diagnosis

Telling Family Members

> *"While Jesus was still speaking, some men came from the house of Jairus, the synagogue ruler. 'Your daughter is dead,' they said. 'Why bother the teacher any more?'"*
> (Mark 5:35)

By now we've already experienced telling loved ones about the diagnosis. Let's look back at some feelings we experienced in handling this situation.

We may recall feeling as though we had let our parents down. Perhaps we felt guilty that we had done something wrong. Remember these are condemning lies from the enemy. He is the king of guilt.

I dreaded telling our parents. I was afraid that my mom would fall to pieces. Again, fear is another of the enemy's weapons. My mom rallied with strength from God. He used her in mighty ways to connect with and minister to other mothers of seriously ill children.

My dad asked me, "What's leukemia?" That was the first time I had to say the "C" word. "It's cancer of the blood, Daddy," I said.

Steve's mom and dad came to the hospital the night of Chad's diagnosis. His mom had a cold and the doctor told us that she couldn't be around Chad until she was well. She came to the door of his room. Steve stepped out into the hallway. I heard her ask without yet knowing the diagnosis, "Can't I see Chad?" I heard Steve say, "No." Then she questioned, "Why not?" Then Steve dropped the bombshell explaining, "Because he can't be around people who are sick because he has cancer." The distraught love of a grandmother was almost unbearable. She looked from the hallway crying as she told him that she loved him and that Mamaw was going to get medicine to get better so that she could see him.

Steve's dad leaned against the wall for physical support. He didn't speak. He was numb. I feared he might collapse.

Although it is never easy to tell a loved one that our child is seriously ill, it is even worse to have a stranger give the news. Unfortunately, that's exactly what happened to Steve's elderly great-aunt, Amy. Our pastor friend, Ira, was on his way to give her the news when a lady who heard the news at a Wednesday night prayer service called her. The lady told Amy that she was so sorry to hear about Chad. Unknowingly, Amy asked her what was wrong with Chad. The lady proceeded to tell Amy that Chad had been diagnosed with cancer.

Later Amy recounted that she felt like she was going to die when she heard the news. Ira arrived within minutes of the phone call and consoled her.

So as difficult as it is to tell a loved one, it is better for them to hear the news from us and not someone else.

17 – Father / Mother

Unite for the Common Cause

> *"Let love and faithfulness never leave you; bind them around your neck, write them on the tablet of your heart. Then you will win favor and a good name in the sight of God and man." (Proverbs 3:3-4)*

No two families are alike. Yet, when a child is diagnosed with a serious illness, there is only one winning and Christ honoring option for parents to choose whether married or divorced: unity.

The distraught love of a grandmother was almost unbearable. She looked from the hallway crying as she told him that she loved him and that Mamaw was going to get medicine to get better so that she could see him.

My friend, Connie, has a godly perspective when it comes to being divorced and being the parent of a seriously ill child. Following her divorce, Connie made the choice that she wanted her daughters to have a right relationship with their father and their new stepmother. She expected the girls to respect and honor the new person in their lives and she expected no less for the girls.

Therefore, after her oldest daughter, Michele, was diagnosed with tongue cancer, Connie chose to continue sharing her daughter. Satan's lie is that we should hold our child closer and tighter, unwilling to share.

When Michele's disease turned from treatment to terminal, Connie honored Michele's request to die at home. She volunteered to move into her ex-husband's family room / basement and cared for Michele until her death. She modeled selfless love.

This brings us to another key topic in parenting a seriously ill child—the essential father. No one can take the place of dad. Whether never married, married, separated, or divorced, dad is a key player in the family, especially of a seriously ill child. Granted, there are extreme situations where some fathers have surrendered their right to be a dad to their family because of sexual abuse, physical abuse, etc. However, other than these extreme situations, the father's role in the illness is vital. Just the presence of a dad says to the child, "You are loved by me" and "I don't care what you look like, I love you for who you are."

> Just the presence of a dad says to the child, "You are loved by me" and "I don't care what you look like, I love you for who you are."

Satan seeks to destroy families. Families wear a target on their backs put there by the enemy. He destroys families by any means. One of the enemy's lies to a dad is about the issue of his manhood. The enemy whispers insults to the father's manhood like, "You deserve to have a 'normal' child" or "Look what you did to your son or daughter." He'll attempt to puncture the pride of a man by making him feel ashamed or embarrassed by the looks of a malformed child. Don't ever forget Satan plays dirty. The truth is that with God's help a dad can be the biggest blessing and encouragement in our child's life.

The father's role is the head of the relationship. The mother's role is the heart and the home of the relationship. When something goes wrong the man wants to "fix it." A father's wiring short circuits when a child is seriously ill. He can't fix it and often feels inadequate or helpless in the situation. Self-esteem may plummet. The enemy's desire is for the father to feel worthless and useless to the family. He may stand on the outskirts watching as the mother tends to and cares for the child. He may walk out silently feeling that he is not needed.

This is another lie from Satan. Satan desires to drive a wedge between the husband and wife. God's truth is that the father holds an essential place in the family. He has the God given task to bring the child "up in the training and instruction of the Lord" (Ephesians 6:5). Our American society has reversed the role. It is common thought that it is the mother's responsibility to teach the children about God. Mothers must pray asking God to reveal ways to draw the father into the center of caring for the seriously ill child. Communicating love during this time is key for the mother and father. At first, the father may have trouble sharing his feelings, especially if this was not role modeled by his father. Patience is essential during this process. Love is faithful and will persevere.

Whether we are the mother or the father, we are helpless in this situation without the hope of Jesus Christ. A pessimistic outlook compounds when the spouse does not have a personal relationship with God. There's earthly hopelessness and eternal hopelessness. To the spouse that may be in such a situation, please continue to love the spouse with Christ-like love and continue to pray for his or her personal relationship with God. God is faithful. It may take years, but God does hear and answer prayer.

If a father is not present, pray for God to provide a father figure. I recall a three year old with cancer who didn't have a father present but did have a grandfather. He was the only father this child had ever known. The child adored his papaw and the feeling was mutual. The saddest of events came when the grandfather was jailed for an unknown reason. The child became terminal. Before the child passed away guards brought the grandfather in shackles to the boy's hospital room to say goodbye.

Beautiful things happen in the family and in the marriage when a father accepts his role as a father of a seriously ill child. A team approach ties and binds the family.

I was blessed to have a husband who accepted his role as a father of a seriously ill child. We worked together as one unit. Steve covered bases at home while I was at the hospital. We didn't have one disagreement while going through the hospital treatments and thereafter. Steve describes it best, "You put you in the background." He said that nothing he could be go-

> Whether we are the mother or the father, we are helpless in this situation without the hope of Jesus Christ.

ing through was half as bad as what Chad was going through.

Steve attends Chad's Individualized Education Plan meetings with me. It pulls great weight for a father to attend meetings. Educators are so used to meeting with only the mother. Chad's kindergarten teacher told us that she doesn't conference with many fathers. There's a definite home team advantage to having a godly dad coaching and cheering his team on. It's a sure prediction for winning.

Those blessed to have a faithful committed spouse must show them how thankful we are for them. In the heat of the battle, it's easy to get discouraged without a word of appreciation.

> Lastly, and of most importance, is the matter of being purposeful to continue intimacy in the relationship.

Lastly, and of most importance, is the matter of being purposeful to continue intimacy in the relationship. This is one of the first areas neglected when caring for the child. However, it is one of the most important areas that needs attention.

Let's make a date with our mate. Take a friend up on their offer to help you. Money may be tight, but a stroll in the park holding hands is free. It is refreshing just to have time to talk.

Also, purposefully plan a "play" date. The key words are "purposefully plan." It may take some creative engineering on our behalf to make this happen. Recall the key word of this devotional is unity. Both need this time to re-connect on a deeper relationship level. This time alone offers us a God—designed way to release the emotions and stress associated with caring for the child. God created this pleasure for the husband and wife. Enjoy it.

18 – The Other Children

What about us?

> *"Adam lay with his wife Eve, and she became pregnant and gave birth to Cain. She said, 'With the help of the Lord I have brought forth a man.' Later she gave birth to his brother Abel. Now Abel kept flocks, and Cain worked the soil." (Genesis 4:1-2)*

Jealousy has existed ever since the first family had the first children. God gifted Cain and Abel with different gifts and talents. He does the same today. Instead of celebrating uniqueness, we become jealous and covet the other person's gifts and talents.

The enemy, the creator of jealousy, whispers lies to us. When another child comes into the family, the older sibling becomes jealous. No longer is he the center of attention. This jealousy is compounded with the sibling of a seriously ill child. The ill child's immediate needs shout for attention as the other child(ren) watch in silence. There are still days when the kids talk about the amount of time I spent with Chad and not with them. We just need to identify it for what it is, jealousy from the enemy, and continue to walk forward.

The healthy child may experience emotions similar to those we as a parent experienced following diagnosis. Their questions may include, "Was it something I did that caused my sibling to be ill?" "Did my wishing he would go away cause this to happen?" They, too, play the blame game.

Parents feel guilt for not being able to give the other child(ren) as much attention as they once did. The enemy is playing the field from both directions. Recognizing the tactic of the enemy is the key to canceling the guilt trip.

Establishing lines of communication early may alleviate some of the guilt and fear the healthy child may be feeling. Katie washed her hands obsessively. They chapped from the numerous washings. Although we reassured her that she couldn't catch cancer from Chad I don't think she really believed us.

A writing from my mother-in-law gives us a picture of Katie and Ryan:

> Katie and Ryan were true warriors thru this.
> They suffered in silence not really knowing what
> they were dealing with. They were separated
> from their parents so much. Little Katie was only
> ten and Ryan six. Katie asked me one night if she
> could catch what Chad had. They always had
> loving grandparents and friends to be with them,
> but nothing could take the place of their parents.

Then the game of life with a seriously ill child begins to play out and the siblings sit on the sidelines and watch. My mother-in-law referred to Katie and Ryan suffering in silence. I have heard so many siblings described that way. They aren't polled before this journey begins. They are hurled into the car along with the parents and the ill child. Dazed and stunned from the change of routine, the healthy child often acts out his neglect. Any change in behavior (such as lashing out in anger) or regression of habits (such as bed-wetting, thumb-sucking, wanting to sleep with mom and dad, etc.) signifies a scream for help.

Establishing lines of communication early may alleviate some of the guilt and fear the healthy child may be feeling.

Also, children take on parent roles. Katie became a sort of "little mother" to Ryan. She watched out for him at school. Helped him with homework. She acted like a little Rita, if you will. During this time she made straight A's. It was all Katie and nothing I was doing to help her. Now she is a beautiful young lady. At times I see a side of Katie that mimics a little girl. It's like all of those years that she missed doing the little girl stuff comes out of her. The way she giggles so carefree. The way she will not stress over much of anything. I'm thankful she is getting to live out a part of her life that she missed.

> Christian counseling is a wonderful investment for a family. We visited a counselor.

Christian counseling is a wonderful investment for a family. We visited a counselor. We saw him as a couple, as an entire family, as the seriously ill child, and as siblings of the seriously ill child.

Chad turned into a terror at the house. He wreaked havoc over Katie and Ryan. I needed some help. Our best counseling session was when the scenario that I had described played out in front of the counselor's eyes. He witnessed the dynamics of our family life and the added resentment that a sick brother who ruled the roost was creating for his brother and sister.

The counselor properly modeled how to handle the situation. I walked out armed with a plan of action of how to handle the situation at home.

Every family struggles with family issues. Our struggles are as unique as our family. Wise Christian counsel can be a healthy way to deal with family struggles. Contact the church for a list of recommended counselors.

With God's help, our family will survive the ride intact.

19 – Home Sweet Home

There's No Place Like Home

> *"When they came to the home of the synagogue ruler, Jesus saw a commotion, with people crying and wailing loudly. He went in and said to them, 'Why all this commotion and wailing? The child is not dead but asleep.' But they laughed at him. After he put them all out, he took the child's father and mother and disciples who were with him, and went in where the child was."*
> (Mark 5:38-40)

I love this story of how Jesus handled the masses and regained a calm, peaceful environment at Jairus' home. He sets the example of home life for those who have a seriously ill child.

The first order of business Jesus took care of was escorting out those who had a negative outlook on the situation—those who were skeptical, those who laughed at him, those who didn't believe him when he told them the girl was only sleeping and not dead.

My friend, Nancy, presents a delicious analogy between being the parent of a seriously ill child and an Oreo cookie:

Most of the time, being a support beam is synonymous with being an Oreo middle. You have the task of holding all ends together, and at the same time, everyone seeks you out to devour you first. Sometimes the devouring comes in the form of asking questions. Sometimes it is merely to provide updates to the masses (which can happen…oh…about 1000 times a week, give or take). Then sometimes it is in the form of receiving news (like test results, good and bad). Being an Oreo middle is important; especially in the beginning of treatment. People aim questions at you like wildfire! Some of these inquiries are valid, considerate, and sensible. The majority of them are stupid, heartless, and unnecessary. Share the information you wish to share. No one has a license to know the details of the treatment plan unless you want them to be privy to this knowledge. So, sometimes it is necessary to protect and proceed with caution. That is when you graduate from Oreo middle to Oreo Double Stuff.

Before we brought Chad home from the hospital we established the Gray House Ground Rules for grandparents. Rule number one: as long as Chad's counts were above a certain number he was allowed visitors. However, please leave your negative thoughts at the door. We said that we knew there would be days that Chad would look like death from the chemo but while they were visiting not one negative thing was to be said. They were welcome to talk at their homes as much as they wished but not at our house.

Next, in dealing with the masses of well-meaning friends, for a while we recorded a daily update on our message machine. We also turned off the ringer so as not to be disturbed. People were welcome to listen and leave us a message, if they wished. Our attention was on Chad and his care.

Obviously, this was before the internet was widely used. Use the internet to your advantage. A distribution list is one way to keep friends and family updated. However, I believe a wise use of your time is to use the free CaringBridgeTM

> Most of the time, being a support beam is synonymous with being an Oreo middle.

> We said that we knew there would be days that Chad would look like death from the chemo but while they were visiting not one negative thing was to be said.

website (www.caringbridge.org). "CaringBridgeTM is a non-profit 501(c)(3) organization offering free personalized Web sites to those wishing to stay in touch with family and friends during significant life events. Their mission is to bring together a global community of care powered by the love of family and friends in an easy, accessible and private way." Their eleven minute video on the website tells the emotional story of how CaringBridgeTM was born.

> Another way to accept the offers from well-meaning friends is to channel them into action outside of your home. If you need errands run, pass them along to those friends.

Another way to accept the offers from well-meaning friends is to channel them into action outside of your home. If you need errands run, pass them along to those friends. So often folks want to help, but they are clueless in exactly how they can help. Give them a task though and they are there for you. Also, try to utilize them in their area of gifts or talents, if you know them. Nothing is more fulfilling for someone with a servant's heart than to serve in a way that allows him to use his gifts and talents.

Steve's great uncle, Bernice, delivered happy meals to Chad when he was in the hospital. Keep in mind he was in his eighties. His son later declared that he wasn't even sure his dad would have known what a happy meal was. But he did, and he didn't miss a day of delivering a happy meal to Chad when he was hospitalized. We didn't ask him to do this. This was his way of saying, "I love you all and I care about you."

Since Chad was in a compromised state with his immune system, visitors were off-limits at the hospital. In the beginning, we were inundated with visits at the hospital. I would step outside of the room to visit for a few minutes. However, it began to take its toll on my mental state of repeating the story over and over. Finally, we put a sign up for visitors on Chad's door where they could write well wishes. That helped slow down traffic.

Upon returning home we were still off-limits to visitors because of Chad's compromised state. This was a blessing in one way because it allowed us to focus on him and rest when he did. By the time our child is diagnosed we are usually physically exhausted. Usually we are up at night with the sick child until he is diagnosed. Then, following diagnosis at the hospital, we all know there is no rest there. It's up and down every night helping the child to the restroom, attending to a beeping pump, and waking to nurses taking vitals.

Our house was visible after rounding a curve. After each hospital stay, when we turned that curve Chad would say,

"Home sweet home" as soon as he saw our house. Home sweet home became an oasis in the desert following diagnosis. It was the place where we set our schedule and did what we wanted to do.

With that new freedom from the hospital came a freedom to establish a new "normal" family routine. Realizing that our family would never again be as we once knew it, freed us to determine the family routine we wanted to have with our new family life. We added the important stuff back onto the calendar like attending church as a family, when counts allowed, and kept off stuff that didn't add value to our family but instead took time away from our family.

20 – Financial Needs

Confess and Swallow Our Pride

> *"Keep your lives free from the love of money and be content with what you have, because God has said, 'Never will I leave you; never will I forsake you.'" (Hebrews 13:5)*

Escalating hospital bills continued to fill the mailbox. Our previous poor money management skills before diagnosis and my current unemployment status were quickly catching up to us. Our finances and my mental state were derailing.

Our electricity payment was due and we had no money to pay it. A refused call to the electric company for financial help left a bitter taste in my mouth.

That afternoon at a red traffic signal, my emotional ditty bag exploded. I verbally cried out to God, "You said you'd never put more on me than I can bear. You must think I'm a lot stronger than I am because I'm about to lose my mind. We're about to go under financially. We don't even have money to pay our electric bill and I don't have any idea where we're going to get it from? Where are you, God?" I questioned sobbing.

That afternoon at a red traffic signal, my emotional ditty bag exploded.

The scripture reference I was grasping for as I cried out to God is 1 Corinthians 10:13 which says, "No temptation has seized you except what is common to man. And God is faithful; he will not let you be tempted beyond what you can bear. But when you are tempted, he will also provide a way out so that you can stand up under it." At the point when I cried out to God with that statement, God knew that my faith in him as my provider was being tempted to turn my back on him, if the need wasn't met. Well, God was faithful to his word.

The electric bill was paid on time and in full. Steve asked his father for help. He paid the bill for us. God humbled us during this time to be willing to accept help from our parents. They paid off Chad's hospital and doctor bills. They bought us groceries. They bought clothes for the children.

God can meet our need any way he chooses. In this case, he humbled me to accept God's way, not mine.

God may choose our parents, neighbors, church family, a non-profit agency, the government, or any other avenue to meet our financial needs. The first step we must take is to admit our need for help. It is our responsibility to speak up when we have a need.

> *The first step we must take is to admit our need for help.*

Romans 12:6-8 speaks about the body of Christ and how each member has different gifts, according to the grace given us. Some have gifts of prophesying, serving, teaching, encouraging, leadership, mercy and contributing to the needs of others. Those gifted with contributing to the needs of others are instructed by the writer of Romans to give generously. God blesses them. They realize their blessings are to be passed on to those in need. When we don't share our needs, we rob others of blessings. When we give, we are blessed, too. Proverbs 11:25 says, "A generous man will prosper; he who refreshes others will himself be refreshed."

21 – Insurance

Learn to Play the Game

> *"But the fruit of the Spirit is love, joy, peace, patience, kindness, goodness, faithfulness, gentleness, and self-control." (Galatians 5:22-23)*

I realize my cross to bear is being the go-between of medical providers and medical insurance providers. Both groups get paid to tell me what else I need to do while I do all of the work for FREE.

I love the writing *What Did You Do All Day?* by Julie J. Gordon, Director of the MUMS National Parent-to-Parent Network. MUMS is a national Parent-to-Parent organization for parents or care providers of a child with any disability, rare or not-so-rare disorder, chromosomal abnormality or health condition. According to Julie, "MUMS' main purpose is to provide support to parents in the form of a networking system that matches them with other parents whose children have the same or similar condition. The MUMS website (www.netnet.net/mums) has a list of disorders. MUMS has parent matches as well as links to support groups for these often rare disorders."

What Did You Do All Day?

By Julie J. Gordon
(Used by permission)

Did you ever sit down after an exhausting day, look around, see a messy house, dishes piled high, laundry overflowing and wonder what did you do all day? Or worse yet, did your husband come home and ask you that same question? You never took a break, sat down and watched TV or read a book, yet you seem to have accomplished nothing all day. Next time you have a thought like this, read the following list and check the ones that apply to you. Perhaps you and your husband and children will be more understanding of the added work a child with special needs can be. Perhaps you will be amazed at all you really did accomplish all day!

THINGS TO DO

- Search Internet for information
- Do range of motion exercises
- Do speech therapy exercises
- Make therapy appointments
- Call in prescriptions for medication
- Call for diapers and supplies to be delivered
- Schedule doctor appointments
- Schedule Home Health Care services
- Call physical therapist for physical therapy services
- Call physical therapist about getting new wheelchair
- Call insurance about wheelchair coverage
- Call Medical Assistance about wheelchair coverage
- Pick out wheelchair
- Order new wheelchair
- Make appointments for wheelchair insert fitting
- Make appointment with orthopedic surgeon
- Set up Respite Care

- Interview & Train new Respite provider
- Make transportation arrangements for Respite
- Pack up child's things for Respite
- Write letter to go with child to Respite
- Call Social Services about reimbursement forms for travel expenses
- Call Social Security Office about income changes
- Call bill collectors about late payments on medical bills
- Call teacher about observing child in classroom
- Observe child at school
- Talk to teacher about Individual Education Program (IEP) changes
- Call school to set up new IEP meeting
- Call advocate to come to IEP meeting
- Meet with advocate
- Call Parent Advocacy group to find out your school rights
- Attend IEP meeting
- Call Special Education Director about unresolved school problems
- Write letter to Department of Public Instruction about unresolved school problems
- Call dentists in town to see who takes Medical Assistance
- Call dentists out of town to see who takes Medical Assistance
- Write letter to legislator about lack of services
- Call hospital about mistake on billing
- Call insurance commissioner about insurance company denials
- Make an appointment to check blood levels
- Schedule another EEG to monitor seizures
- Call school about doctor appointments
- Call bus company not to pick up child on appointment days
- Call baby-sitter for other children for appointments

- Bring child to doctor appointments
- Go for communication evaluation
- Call around to see who pays for computers
- Write letter justifying computer
- Call therapists to write letter about computer
- Teach self & child to use computer
- Set up orthodontics (braces) appointments
- Bring child to have leg braces made
- Bring child to have leg braces adjusted
- Call around looking for a van to buy
- Call everyone to see who can help with van expenses
- Set up Community Options Program Assessment
- Call Family Support Program for help with expenses
- Call and compare prices of van lifts
- Call everyone about help with lift costs
- Write letter justifying lift
- Look at vans and buy one
- Go to Bank for loan for van and fill out forms
- Make an appointment for lift installation
- Bring van for lift installation
- Pick up forms at Social Services
- Go to Social Security for SSI reevaluation
- Go to therapeutic swim class
- Write list of child's care needs
- Train Home Health Provider
- Pick up prescriptions
- Fill out Katie Becket MA waiver forms
- Fill out Family Support forms
- Fill out Respite Care forms
- Make communication board
- Teach child how to use communication board
- Attend School Board meeting
- Attend support group meetings
- Take child in for blood levels
- Take child for EEG

- Have COP assessment in home
- Meet with Home Health Care nurse
- Pay numerous medical bills
- Research Hyperbaric Oxygen Therapy (HBOT)
- Have fund-raiser
- Second mortgage house
- Take child for Hyperbaric Oxygen Therapy (HBOT)
- Write letter or e-mail to MUMS for help!!!!!!!!!

"None of these things show at the end of a busy day. All of these things are important and take a lot of time. Some of them you do once in a while and some on a regular basis. Make your own list so you can see for yourself (and those who ask) how your time is spent. Add to this list those things other parents must do such as: grocery shopping, cooking, volunteering at schools, bringing car in for repairs, cleaning, laundry, etc. If you are a mother working outside the home too—How do you do it???????"

Julie's writing helps us see that making calls to an insurance claims representative or to a medical providers' insurance department is a part of the big picture of caring for our child. My medical insurance activity has downsized. I now dedicate one half day usually every two weeks to make phone calls to a claims representative or to a medical providers' insurance department.

I don't ever see myself out of a job as the go between for insurance and medical providers. It's God's way of maturing my fruits of the Spirit. Thank you, God, for insurance.

22 – The Diagnosis

What Do We Tell Our Child?

"Love does not delight in evil but rejoices with the truth."
(1 Corinthians 13:6)

Dr. K asked, "Have you told Chad yet?" "No," I said, "What do I tell him?" "Do you want me to tell him?" he questioned. "Yes," I replied quickly.

Dr. K said, "Chad you have sick blood. We're going to give you special medicine to make your blood better."

Chad replied, "Okay."

In looking back over that conversation, two ideas grab my attention. First, about how simple the explanation was and secondly, about how trusting Chad was. That's the innocence of a preschooler. As we age, we lose our innocence. However, children with life-threatening illnesses are robbed of that innocence.

Along with our own feelings of anger, guilt, and fear, we also experience feelings of overwhelming love and protectiveness. We may be tempted not to tell our child about his diagnosis. There's a part of our heart that doesn't want our child to have to deal with this disease. We don't want our child's innocence stolen away by a disease that no one should ever have to endure.

However, not verbalizing it to our child does not change the facts. Every child, no matter what age, knows when something is not right. The clues are obvious. First, the child is sleeping at the hospital instead of at home. Strangers in white coats parade into the room. The child doesn't feel well. People are whispering and talking in secretive code.

Choosing not to tell the child shuts down communication instead of encouraging open communication. The child knows something is going on and is forced to protect the parent by not talking about the subject. If the child can't talk to us, then he will either talk to someone else about his feelings or just harmfully bury them. He will have questions just like we did when we received the diagnosis—Why me? Did I do something wrong? We want to be the person answering these questions with God giving us wisdom and strength. Don't let another person have the responsibility God has entrusted to us, and certainly do what you can to help him to not bury his feelings.

If communication has been a struggle in the past, let's vow this day that we will put forth our best effort with God's help to change that. "It's always been like this and it always will be," is a lie from the enemy. Not only does he desire to rob us of joy in the past, but of future joy, too. The enemy wants to create an atmosphere of distrust between the parent and the child. Remember he's all about the business of wrecking families. We are his number one threat. He hates a God-centered loving family. Friend, with God's help we can break any vicious cycle or habit of the past.

Although the disease is painful, the outcome is unsure, and our child has been robbed of his innocence, be assured that there are certain things this disease cannot do. A friend

> Every child, no matter what age, knows when something is not right.

gave this poem to me. I never tire of being reminded of the truth it speaks. Fill the name of your child's disease, injury or birth defect in the parentheses.

What (Cancer) Cannot Do
[Unknown Author]

(Cancer) is so limited…

It cannot cripple love,

It cannot shatter hope,

It cannot corrode faith,

It cannot destroy peace,

It cannot kill friendship,

It cannot suppress memories,

It cannot silence courage,

It cannot invade the soul,

It cannot steal eternal life,

It cannot conquer the spirit

23 – The Prognosis

I Might Die. If I Die Will You Go with Me?

> *"There is a time for everything, and a season for every activity under heaven: a time to be born and a time to die, a time to plant and a time to uproot" (Ecclesiastes 3:1-2)*

Chad looked up at me from his hospital bed and said straight forwardly, "I might die. If I die will you go with me?"

Only five days after being diagnosed with "sick blood," Chad looked up at me from his hospital bed and said straight forwardly, "I might die. If I die will you go with me?" Children have the ability to speak truth in a heart-piercing manner. His three-word statement and question cut through all of my raw emotions and went to the very heart of the issue of Chad's cancer—that children die from cancer—that my child might die from cancer.

I wanted to avoid the issue. I purposefully chose not to say the "C" word in front of Chad. We allowed no one to mention death or dying, yet he still knew. He knew and openly admitted something I didn't want to.

Unprepared and unwilling to go to the land of death and dying, I did not answer. I cried and prayed over the response I would give when his question re-surfaced.

I soon discovered all children think about dying. The diagnosis of cancer only pushes that concept closer to the front of their minds.

God was good to me. He allowed me time to formulate an honest answer to Chad's initial question. Almost two years passed before Chad's question re-surfaced. "Am I going to die?" he asked one day as we were traveling home. Rehearsed and ready, I replied, "Yes, Chad, one day you will die, just as one day I will die. According to Ecclesiastes 3:2 everyone has a time to be born and a time to die. What is most important is that you know that when you die, you will 'be there,' you will be in heaven."

His reply was a trusting, "Okay."

Later that year, Chad prayed to receive Christ as his Savior. He made the promise to "be there," in heaven whenever his time to die should come.

We did not realize the extent Chad was thinking about death until almost four and a half years after his diagnosis. One day in English, Chad's thoughts accidentally spilled out during a writing prompt:

> SUBJECT: *Think about a time when you felt out of place. Write a brief paragraph telling how you felt, why you felt that way, and what you did to feel better.*

Chad's response: "While I was going through my chemotherapy treatments, I did not have hair. It fell out by the handfuls. My dad had hair and I did not. I felt hopeless. I felt hopeless because I thought I was going to die. I trided[sic] my hardest to stay alive by praying. Everywhere I went, I wore a hat."

Do you see how he attempted to cover up the real hopelessness? I helped him with this writing prompt. He wanted to be finished after the "I felt hopeless" sentence. I asked the next question—"Why did you feel hopeless?" It was then that he honestly shared his thoughts about dying. This seven-sentence paragraph written by a ten-year-old speaks volumes about many adult areas of life: feelings, coping skills, serious illness, death, prayer, and hope through Jesus Christ. Chad is truly older than his years in many areas of his life. This is what I mean by being robbed of childhood innocence.

Again, in another writing prompt in October 2003, now seven years since diagnosis, Chad wrote this: "I understand that I will die someday. I say I will not be here long. I dream

We did not realize the extent Chad was thinking about death until almost four and a half years after his diagnosis.

to live a long life. I hope to get out of school. I am a talented guy that likes to play basketball."

Your child may not be as vocal as Chad was. Some children are simply too young. Others simply may not be willing to verbally express their concerns about dying. There are play therapists that can be helpful with less vocal children. A play therapist gives a child a piece of paper and asks the child to draw a picture of anything. The child may draw a picture and then place a single balloon floating to the sky. This balloon may represent the child. The child intuitively knows that death is inevitable.

Perhaps your child has initiated a similar question. Were you prepared to answer your child's question? If your child has not yet asked you this question, how will you answer it when it is presented to you?

God will enable us to talk about the subject when it arises, if we will only ask him for his help.

24 – Attitude with a Capital A

The Strong Willed Child Takes on Life-Threatening Illness

"'Who of you by worrying can add a single hour to his life?'" (Matthew 6:27)

Chad's 5th birthday photo shows a pale skinned boy wearing a plastic yellow construction "hard hat" hiding his bald head with a snarled up lip and a look in his eyes that says, "Cancer, hit me with your best shot. I don't think you can take me."

Once he got the death issue off of his chest, he resigned himself to attacking leukemia the same way he had approached everything else in his four short years of life: head-on with the vengeance of a strong-willed child. He was born a strong-willed child. I thought Ryan was strong-willed until Chad came along. Now Ryan is natured like a couch potato whom we check periodically for a pulse. The joke around the house is that we have a couch tator and an agitator.

Chad is the preschooler who when asked at 3 a.m. by the admitting nurse if he wanted anything to eat replied, "Beans."

These children seem to respond so well to this rigorous challenge because they will not bargain with it.

And yet, it is this tenacious will that seems to help children fight something that is so much bigger than they are. These children seem to respond so well to this rigorous challenge because they will not bargain with it. They step up to the challenge and give it the fight of their lives.

Children live for the present and for themselves. The world revolves around them. That's the way God made them to think. Therefore, unlike adults, they don't sit around worrying, "What's next?" or "What if?" Their concern is "What's now?" This is not to say that they don't think about death and dying, they just don't allow it a prominent space in their thoughts. They give much more thought to living.

Chad didn't fret when he was to go back to the hospital for his next treatment. At the end of each treatment, he walked out of the hospital and didn't look back. It was just like he had done that for the day. He was on a mission to move onto what was next on his list to do for the day. It always involved playing and eating french fries.

> At the end of each treatment, he walked out of the hospital and didn't look back.

This attitude is a gift from God. Steve said that he didn't get upset because Chad didn't get upset. He said if Chad had cried a lot and fought the treatments all of the time it would have been so painful to bear. That's not to say that it wasn't a horrid disease to fight. It was, but Chad's attitude kept us emotionally strong. *How could we wimp out if he wasn't?*

My friend Nancy observed that children believe what parents tell them. She said that she overheard parents say to their children, "Lie down, you're sick." She asked, "What are we telling these kids?" Her attitude with her son, Ryan, was "Get out of bed, you're not sick." If you don't see your child working with a "What's next?" mentality, I encourage you to take the initiative to plan some "What's next?" things for your child to look forward to doing.

25 – Loneliness

Where are Our Child's Friends?

> *"Rejoice with those who rejoice; mourn with those who mourn." (Romans 12:15)*

In kindergarten Chad wanted a friend so badly. I received a phone call from a boy's mother inviting Chad over for a play date. Chad had a wonderful time. He talked fondly of all the fun things he did.

Then I received another phone call from the boy's mother. She began by talking about how active Chad was and that she was afraid he was going to hurt himself. She continued on saying that she didn't feel it would be good for Chad and her son to become friends because she was afraid Chad would die and that she didn't want her son to have to deal with that. I won't share the thoughts that went through my mind as she freely expressed her concerns for her son. I took the high road and graciously bowed out of any friendships with her son.

That afternoon I picked Chad up from school. Beaming with excitement, he asked when he and his new friend could get together for another play date. I explained that his mom didn't think it would be a good idea to continue the friendship. He dropped his head and his pitiful hurt heart said, "He doesn't like me." "Oh no, Baby. It's not that at all." I assured him while wiping tears from my cheeks, "There's nothing not to like about you. You are a great friend." I stroked his cotton soft new growth of hair. "It's his loss, not yours."

That was the first heart-wrenching lesson I learned about my children establishing friendships, we play on our turf first. In fact, we have a family policy. Our home is always open because then we know where our children are, whom they are with, and what they are into.

The second lesson I learned about my children establishing friendships is that sometimes the best friends have four legs. They love at all times. They don't worry about the future because they're not human.

Sometimes the best friends have four legs. They love at all times. They don't worry about the future because they're not human.

We couldn't have a dog during the intensive treatments because of Chad's low counts. Dr. K had a Boston Terrier named Daisy. He talked to Chad about Daisy. Chad would ask Dr. K about Daisy during every hospital stay. Daisy's pictures graced the clinic walls along with the pictures of Dr. K's "children."

However, on the day of Chad's bone marrow check at the end of the intensive treatments, Dr. K. told Chad, "Great news, Chad. Your bone marrow looks great. You are finished with these hospital treatments. You are going onto the maintenance phase." Still under the influence of the anesthesia in a groggy voice, Chad asked, "Dr. K, can I have a Daisy dog now?" Without any consent and without so much as a glance at mom for approval, Dr. K popped, "Yes, Chad. You may have a Daisy dog now."

Excuse me! No one consulted with the mom! I wanted to shout. It was too late. The conspiracy had begun.

That Saturday Chad wanted to go to the pet store to look at fish. "Okay we'll look at fish," I thought.

What I didn't expect was Chad's favorite chemo nurse, Melissa, and her daughter to be at the store. As soon as Melissa saw Chad she enthusiastically said, "Chad, come over here. You've got to see this puppy over here. It's the cutest thing!" The local animal shelter had dogs available for adoption.

"Hold on here! No. No," I was saying, but no one was listening. They'd all gone to look at the puppy.

It was too late. The conspiracy was complete. The doctor and nurse had ganged up on me. I didn't stand a prayer.

We walked out with a girl Border Collie mix puppy, white with red markings. The kids named her Missy, which is fitting as I later learned that is what Melissa's brothers call her.

I agree, though, that a dog is man's best friend. She has brought each family member joy, especially Chad. She's always available to give you a wet kiss on your cheek. She wags her tail to say, "I love you just the way you are."

26 – Late-Effect Emotions

Dormant Emotions Erupt After the Crisis

"Devote yourselves to prayer, being watchful and thankful."
(Colossians 3:19)

"Nobody ever told us that the emotions don't end with the crisis. It's reassuring to know that we didn't do anything wrong and that it's not abnormal to have these emotional aftermaths, years after the crisis is past." A mother shared these words about her teenager who was born with a life-threatening birth defect. She continued, "We can recognize it for what it is— the ugly today wasn't caused by today but by what has been brewing for how many years." It's like a dormant volcano erupting years after the last explosion.

"This is a teenager who never got to be a child. Now instead of expressing teenage emotions he is expressing emotions as a child since he never got to be a child during the childhood years. This teenager doesn't know how to process decisions about high school and other things because he never thought he would live to see high school."

"Then there are the siblings," she added. "They had to be more than they were during the crisis and now they too are dealing with emotions that are stemming from the crisis years after the fact."

This may best be described as toxic ash from an active volcano. "And yet we can't excuse it but must continue to deal with emotions that might be inappropriate for the current age but are right on target for someone who was deprived of living his actual age when he went through the crisis." Instead, he lived adulthood first by dealing with issues like death and

> "We can recognize it for what it is— the ugly today wasn't caused by today but by what has been brewing for how many years."

having countless procedures and treatments usually reserved for those who have lived a long, productive life.

As if the teen years aren't turbulent enough. The equation says adolescence equals change—physical, social, cognitive and spiritual change. Compound on that a teen that missed the physical, social, cognitive and spiritual change of his childhood years.

Just like a volcano, we may notice warning signs of a possible future eruption. Short negative comments, a disgruntled spirit (nothing is right), and even the body language may be those small warning signs to a parent that a dangerous eruption could be coming. As parents, immersion in prayer during these warning signs is critical to minimizing the amount of damage when the teen explodes. Open lines of communication continue to be vital.

It's a question of timing. *When will the teen explode?* There may be an external factor (a move, changing schools, changing churches, etc.) that prompts the eruption or it may be an internal factor. Those are more difficult to recognize. Growth spurts are an outward indicator of all of the internal changes taking place in the teen's body. Emotions swell in all teens. However, the additional past adult experiences of the teen that faced and survived a life-threatening illness in childhood, silently play into this equation exponentially. A sound or a smell may trigger a painful memory buried deep within the crevices of his mind. Whatever the trigger may be, that is all it takes to expose the raw underlying emotions for the teen.

At that point, put your dust mask on. The explosion spews miserable ash onto the observers standing by, once again, the parents and the siblings. Ash is the nuisance that reminds everyone, everyday that an active volcano smolders nearby. A serious ashing can make life miserable for all living within spewing distance. Air quality around the volcano is vital to the health and well being of all living near the volcano.

Sometimes the volcano also explodes inwardly as well as outwardly. I have one friend who has a daughter who is doing self-destructive things to her body like purging herself after meals. Another friend has a daughter who was a sibling of a teen girl who passed away. This girl turned inwardly and outwardly. She would physically attack friends with her fingernails. She also turned inwardly by purging herself.

Don't forget those who are just visiting near the volcano but have limited or no prior knowledge of the volcano's past.

> Short negative comments, a disgruntled spirit (nothing is right), and even the body language may be those small warning signs to a parent that a dangerous eruption could be coming.

Be on guard not to allow teachers, friends and parents of friends, church family, or even neighbors to be so quick to judge the eruptions of the volcano. Too often these people compound the problem by adding labels to the teen. No additional labels are needed. This teen has already had enough unusual labels.

As much as the dormant emotions of a teen can be compared to a dormant volcano, God's truth is that this is his child that he created in his image. He loves this teen. As this teen's #1 cheerleader, our responsibilities continue to be to love this teen, to pray for this teen, and to continue to talk to this teen. Again, with God's wisdom and knowledge speaking to you through the Holy Spirit, he will prick your heart to know exactly what is the best approach in helping your teen continue to walk through this area of the crisis. It won't be easy. Nothing has been so far for this teen. That's the enemy's plan. He's still on his mission to steal, kill and destroy.

Our counter-attack is to stay on our knees seeking God's heart on behalf of our children, no matter what their ages. Also, in both cases the parents of the girls took a very aggressive approach to getting help in the situation. They enlisted prayer partners to pray for the parents and the teen. Also, they made close friends and relatives aware of the situation so they too could hold the teen accountable regarding the purging. God brought both of them through the crisis.

> Our counter-attack is to stay on our knees seeking God's heart on behalf of our children, no matter what their ages.

27 – God has a Plan and a Purpose for Our Child

Helping Our Child Discover His Purpose

"Before I formed you in the womb I knew you, before you were born I set you apart; I appointed you as a prophet to the nations." (Jeremiah 1:5)

Jeremiah received his purpose to be a prophet from God before he was born. So when Jeremiah uses the excuse that he can't speak because he is only a child, God quickly reminds him, "Do not say, 'I am only a child.' You must go to everyone I send you to and say whatever I command you. Do not be afraid of them, for I am with you and will rescue you" (Jeremiah 1:7-8).

Age doesn't matter to God. He starts with everyone at the same time in his or her life, before conception. God is thinking about us and has a plan and purpose for us before we take our first breath.

God creates each creature uniquely. No one will ever be like you. Therefore, there is no one else who can do the job God created you to do for him. We were created to serve God through serving others.

The same is true for our child. He is gifted with certain gifts and talents that no one else has in order to serve God in a way that no one else can.

I love to watch God work the puzzle of life. It's always an "Ah ha" moment when God allows me to see how he has been orchestrating situations behind the scenes to bring his plan to be. He is a great God!

Meet Jean Driscoll. The Bible verse she claims is John 17:4, "I have brought you glory on earth by completing the work you gave me to do." Being born with spina bifida didn't deter Jean from pursuing God's plan and purpose for her life. In her autobiography *Determined to Win: The Overcoming Spirit of Jean Driscoll*, Terry Meeuwsen accurately states about Jean's journey through life, "But for Jean Driscoll every accomplishment, from the moment of birth to her eighth Boston Marathon trophy, was won only after overcoming discouragement, frustration, pain, and disappointment. She is living proof that the only limitations that can keep us down are in our hearts and minds." That's why this champion in life encouraged Chad at the 2005 Maryland/Delaware State Fellowship of Christian Athletes' Victory Celebration Banquet to "Dream BIG!" That is Jean's motto.

Jean is a world-class athlete, Olympian, author, motivational speaker and advocate worldwide for persons with disabilities. She has also done work as a television sports commentator and is the co-founder of a non-profit organization called Determined to Win.

Jean has won the Boston Marathon eight times and is the only person in history to achieve that feat. She is an Olympic athlete who won silver medals in the 1992 and 1996 Summer Olympic Games. She is also a world record holder in the 10,000-meter track event as well as the 10K and marathon road racing distances. Sports Illustrated for Women recognizes Jean as one of the top 25 female athletes of the twentieth century.

Jean periodically coaches at wheelchair track camps during the summer. She is also working in the field of health care. She does Electro Dermal Screening, a type of Biofeedback.

> I love to watch God work the puzzle of life.

She recently traveled to Ghana, West Africa with Joni and Friends for her third time. She worked with the Ghanaian wheelchair athletes and had opportunities to meet with Ghanaian officials to talk about people with disabilities in their country. Check out her website at www.jeandriscoll.com.

28 – Sharing God with Your Child

Do You Know the Great Physician?

> *"They begged him to let them touch even the edge of his cloak, and all who touched him were healed." (Mark 6:56)*

The first step to introducing your child to Jesus is to know him yourself.

I was struck with awe as I rounded the semi-circle hallway and entered the administration building of a world-renowned hospital in Baltimore, Maryland. I was humbled by the massive sculpture. The ten-and-a-half-foot-high sculpture of Jesus cut from a single block of Carrara marble took nine years to complete. Scripture carved at the base reminds me that Jesus is the tender loving comforter as well as healer of my soul. "Come to me, all you who are weary and burdened, and I will give you rest." Matthew 11:28 beckons us to bring our smallest concern to him in order to find true rest in his tender loving arms. Jesus' outstretched arms bids all that pass by to come to him.

The carved feet are smooth and shiny from the touch of passers-by. Bouquets of flowers, coins and writings lie at his feet.

Steve and I touched the massive feet. Looking at me with tear filled eyes he said, "That's where we're supposed to leave all of our cares—at the feet of the Divine Healer."

My eyes scroll up to Jesus' hands. In each palm is a scar from the nails he bore on the cross in order to bring divine healing for my sin.

We all have sin in our lives. We are born with it. It eats away at us and ravages our body, mind and soul. If left untreated it brings eternal punishment to our soul. Fortunately, God freely gave us the cure for our sin through his son's blood. Jesus Christ died on the cross for all sin. All we must do is accept his gift of healing and be cured of the penalty of our sin. I accepted God's healing for my sin on October 16, 1972. On September 23, 1999, Chad prayed to the Great Physician and accepted his free gift of healing for his sin. Our

> Jesus Christ died on the cross for all sin. All we must do is accept his gift of healing and be cured of the penalty of our sin.

family's eternal circle was completed with that decision. Praise the Lord!

Near the carved sculpture, two lecterns hold journals of rule lined paper filled with testaments to the physical, emotional and spiritual healing that innumerable visitors have experienced as they have come to know Jesus, the Great Physician. A framed picture of the sculpture hangs above the journal I signed. The words "Divine Healer" are engraved under the picture. I ponder what words would be worthy to write to Jesus, my tender loving comforter. "Thank you for healing Chad. Love, Chad's Mom."

29 – Miracles, Faith, Hope, and Healing

"Now faith is being sure of what we hope for and certain of what we do not see." (Hebrews 11:1)

"The Other Side of Zero", Part 1

By Nancy Brown

Miracles

Getting pregnant was not an easy task for me. We tried to begin our family the traditional way. I remember sporadically falling to my knees during the "I might be pregnant right now" stages of my cycle and begging God for the miracle. As it turned out, my quest for a baby of my own would require a few attempts at in vitro fertilization. After two failed attempts at conceiving, we came upon our third try to make a baby. On the day we were to find out if all of our efforts (medications, surgery, patience, prayer, etc.) had paid off, I chickened out of hearing the news firsthand. The doctor had phoned me on two separate occasions to "let me down easy" and I just could not bear to hear this knowing that I might be unable to try to get pregnant again. On April 10, 1995, JJ came home with the news. I would be a Mommy after all. I got my miracle.

Nancy affectionately refers to Ryan as her "special egg. The one that hatched." Early in Nancy's pregnancy she discovered she was carrying twins. Sadly, she miscarried the other baby during the first trimester.

"I thank God for 'the miracle named Ryan' everyday."

Faith, Hope, and Healing

You don't realize how together your life is until it all falls apart. My world crumbled on the chilly night of February 9,

You don't realize how together your life is until it all falls apart.

1999. My point of view comes from the pains, perils, and triumphs of being the parent of a cancer kid.

Through my shock and tears, I thought, How could and why would God give this child to me only to take him away?

Each night for the next ten days of testing brought more bad news. The tumor biopsy showed that we were definitely dealing with a malignancy. The bone marrow biopsy confirmed that the disease had metastasized to the bone marrow. The bone scan showed that Ryan had disease in at least three areas of his bones including his skull, his jaw, and his hip/backbone areas.

I began to think that Ryan was beyond help. I became so depressed that I flew down to the computer and, between sobs, I pounded out a letter to each living person I knew requesting prayers for Ryan to recover. I think I really took his doctor by surprise when I asked her to throw in a prayer if she could. All of the information at this stage of the game pointed to a poor recovery. I thought all hope had been lost, so I decided to give the solution to God. I felt that this was the only way my family would survive.

The next day we were awaiting the results of the MIBG scan. This would make it or break it (even though the situation seemed out of control to begin with). As Dr. M, the woman that I hated just for having the unfortunate job of being the messenger, entered the room, the sun shone from behind her, and she looked like an angel. She won my heart and implicit trust when she said, with a broad smile on her face, "the MIBG showed no surprises. We know what to do." It suddenly became so clear to me—I had prayed to God for Ryan to be healed. Here was my answer. Dr. M was sent by God to help him fix this problem.

I had prayed and wondered why this cancer had to touch Ryan. In the split second it took for Dr. M to enter the room and "earn her wings," I began to realize the profound effect that one person can have on the life of another. It was then that the thought dawned on me. If one person could have such a positive affect on another's life, could the reverse be true? Could I inadvertently be poisoning Ryan's mind against becoming healthy again? Even a three-year-old can pick up on negative thoughts and feelings; perhaps even more so than an adult. I made a quick but heartfelt decision at this point. First of all, I would entrust the care of my child to God and to the doctors. After all, they know what they are doing. Second of all, I would commit myself to being a positive and

> As Dr. M, the woman that I hated just for having the unfortunate job of being the messenger, entered the room, the sun shone from behind her, and she looked like an angel.

comforting force in Ryan's life. I would be his cheerleader throughout this long haul.

Since this revelation, I have not shed another tear about this cancer. I have cried happy tears when I heard stories of recovery and hope, but I refused to dwell upon anything that did not apply. It would all be fine. I was sure of that. All I had to do was figure out a way to make this time in Ryan's life seem normal. All I had to do was make cancer an adventure.

Miracles Follow-up

Ryan completed his protocol that included a bone marrow transplant. He is in complete remission. His side effects from his course of treatments include hearing loss, heart damage and reduced pulmonary function. Hearing aids compensate for the hearing loss and a pill for the heart damage. A follow-up cardiologist appointment revealed another miracle. The cardiologist said, "I can't explain this but his heart is normal." Thank you God for "the miracle named Ryan" and for once again healing him.

30 – Everything in Life Can't Be Fun

"Praise the Lord, O my soul, and forget not all his benefits—who satisfies your desires with good things so that your youth is renewed like the eagle's." (Psalm 103:2,5)

"The Other Side of Zero", Part 2

By Nancy Brown

Growing up, Nancy's mother told her, "Everything in life can't be fun." Accepting that statement as a challenge, Nancy made it her mission to prove her mother wrong.

Remember, cancer is as big as you make it. It already took up 75% of our lives. I refused to let it take the days out of the hospital, too.

One of the most costly side-effects of this whole cancer experience has been the loss of childhood that Ryan endured. This has been the worst part. For all the time that Ryan should have been at the playground with his friends, he was in the playroom of the inpatient unit wearing a surgical mask to prevent any germs from entering his body. When he should have been at the pool pushing inflatable beach balls over the top of the water, he was walking the halls of the hospital pushing an IV pole around. The times he should have been enjoying birthday parties and holidays, he was receiving

When he should have been at the pool pushing inflatable beach balls over the top of the water, he was walking the halls of the hospital pushing an IV pole around.

chemotherapy. While his friends were pushing each other on the swing set, Ryan was in isolation because he was unable to be in the mainstream of society as immunodepressed as he was. This was not easy, but I still attempted to make all of this part of our adventure.

I invented "chemo camp." This is what we called our three to four day stays in the hospital for chemotherapy. For this event, we had special bedding. He opted for the red, purple, turquoise, and green dinosaur sheets and comforter. To put it mildly, when Ryan was hospitalized, everyone could find his room. When an accident occurred on the sheets and they needed laundering, everyone knew to whom the drying load belonged. We also hung up window clings, and brought some favorite toys from home.

Neutropenia camp, which usually lasted several days more than chemo camp, involved many of the same things. The only difference is that our activity level was restricted. During chemo camp or a blood transfusion, Ryan was not permitted to leave the 8th floor. At any other time, the hospital was our oyster, so to speak. We would walk the halls, with IV pole in tow. To make camp more fun, we invented what Ryan called "ski-watering." This involved Ryan standing on the IV pole base with me pushing him around the place as quickly as he could tolerate. We wheelchair raced, went to the admissions area fish tank (which we called "the aquarium") and spent a considerable time in the hospital gift shop.

I usually tried to have Ryan make at least one trip out of his room on a daily basis no matter what his condition. Call me a torture chamber operator, but I believe heavily in the theory that a change of scenery can do wonders for the soul (even if this change of scenery is another part of a hospital). It seemed to work best on days when it took more effort. Quite frankly, there were days when all of the effort was mine.

I usually tried to have Ryan make at least one trip out of his room on a daily basis no matter what his condition.

Ryan had everyone wrapped around his little finger by the time his bone marrow transplant rolled around. All of the nurses had his routine down pat, and he had no problem being the guy in charge. Ryan always made sure that his needs were known. He went from not speaking to anyone in the beginning of treatment to basically ruling the roost. His nicknames at the hospital were "Downtown Ryan Brown" and "the Mayor." He lived up to both names well.

Chad also became comfortable with the staff and facilities. One day a resident came into examine Chad. The doctor said, "Hello, I'm Dr. B." and Chad said, "Hello, I'm Dr.

Chadwinsky." Keep in mind that the Chief of Pediatric Hematology/Oncology was Dr. Kalwinsky. The room rolled in laughter.

Be sure to file laughter in the main "crisis" folder. Refer back to laughter when addressing the subheadings. The subheadings include any area of the crisis that is not fun.

> Another rule of thumb is "less is more." Talking about the crisis only draws more attention to it.

Another rule of thumb is "less is more." Talking about the crisis only draws more attention to it. Chad taught me this lesson during swimming lessons. He still had his Hickman catheter. I covered it with a clear plastic covering called a Tegaderm which sort of vacuum wrapped "Buddy," Chad's nickname for his catheter.

We hadn't pulled out of the parking space after the first lesson when Chad announced, "Julia asked me about Buddy." "She did?" I questioned. "Yes, she said, 'What's that?'" he said.

I began the teachable moment. "Did you explain to her who Buddy is? That he is your friend and as long as you have Buddy you don't have to have ouchies in your arm for blood work?" I asked.

"No," Chad replied. "Well, did you tell her that you had sick blood and this is how you get your medicine to help make your blood better?" I questioned.

"No," Chad replied again. By now I'm wondering what in the world he has told her and what I'm going to say when I get a phone call from her parents.

"Chad, exactly what did you say to Julia when she asked you what Buddy was?" I questioned, almost dreading to hear his answer.

He said, "I told her, 'You don't even want to know.'" The quick wit of my son was priceless. I burst into laughter. Chad was not asked another question that week.

By the time you're through the crisis you should have a file folder brimming over with laughter.

31 – Two Wonderful Things Our Children Deserve to Experience

Wishes and Camp

> *"Dear Friend, I pray that you may enjoy good health and that all may go well with you, even as your soul is getting along well." (3 John 1:2)*

Wishes

"Your child is well deserving," Dr. D said firmly when I questioned her about Chad having a wish granted. I realize that lots of parents are offered the option soon after diagnosis. However, Chad was not. I mistakenly thought wishes were reserved for children whom the doctor thought were going to die. So it was perfectly okay with me that Dr. K didn't offer Chad the opportunity to have a wish granted.

When I shared with our Richmond doctor that we were going to the world-renowned family theme park in Florida. She asked, "You're going through a wish foundation aren't you?"

"No," was my response. Following some very pointed questions she set the record straight. "Wishes are for any child with a life-threatening illness," she explained. She said that early on wishes were reserved for children who only had a high risk factor. She went on to say that Chad would have been eligible because he did have a high risk factor. Her mission was to change my negative thoughts about wishes.

Following Chad's exam, the social worker came in with a brochure and the business card of the local chapter of a national wish-granting foundation, Make-A-Wish Foundation® of America (www.wish.org).

Steve called and learned the specifics about wishes they do and do not grant. He learned that, "Most wish requests fall into four major categories:

1. **I wish to go**

   Some Make-A-Wish kids want to travel to their favorite theme park, while others want to visit an exotic beach, go on a cruise, see snow for the first time, or attend a major sporting event or concert.

2. **I wish to be**

   Children search the depths of their imagination when they wish to be someone for a day—a fireman, a police officer, or a model, for instance.

3. **I wish to meet**

   Many want to meet their favorite athlete, recording artist, television personality, movie star, politician, or public figure.

4. I wish to have

Children often wish for a special gift, like a computer, a tree house, a shopping spree, or something that they have coveted for a long time."

In 2005, Make-A-Wish Foundation celebrated its 25th Anniversary. Since 1980, Make-A-Wish Foundation's mission has been to "grant the wishes of children with life-threatening medical conditions to enrich the human experience with hope, strength, and joy."

We waited six months before approaching Chad about a wish. Finally, I concluded that I was allowing the enemy to steal Chad's future joy by believing his lie that only children who are going to die have wishes granted.

We brought the subject up at the dinner table. We thought Chad might have trouble thinking of what to wish for. We must have been delirious. A child that doesn't know what to wish for? Yeah. Right!

We started out the conversation by asking, "Chad if you could have any wish, what would it be?" Expecting hesitancy or the need for suggestions, we waited.

Immediately, he burst with excitement, "I'd ask for a swimming pool." My mouth dropped in disbelief. How long had he been thinking about this? Steve informed him that the Make-A-Wish Foundation® does not grant wishes for swimming pools, and then asked, "So what's your second wish?"

Chad said thoughtfully, "Then, I wish to see a whale."

Two wish volunteers interviewed Chad. After some discussion, Chad told them that he wanted to see the whales and to swim with the dolphins.

The wish office worked with us to determine a time that would fit with our schedule. Within a couple of weeks Chad was on his way to Florida to "see the whales and to swim with the dolphins."

If you have reservations about allowing your child to have a wish granted, I encourage you to release any lie the enemy has been whispering to you and allow your child to experience one of the most memorable moments in his life.

Our family was treated like royalty beginning with the limousine ride from our home and ending with the drop off to our home, again by limousine. Everything in between was a dream come true, even for adults.

The highlight of the trip was seeing Chad's face the first

The highlight of the trip was seeing Chad's face the first time he saw the whale show and when he stepped into the water to have his personal dolphin encounter. In fact, Chad was the first national wish child to go to this dolphin theme park. You can read Chad's wish story that I wrote at www.wish.org/home/wishes_go_chad.htm.

time he saw the whale show and when he stepped into the water to have his personal dolphin encounter.

This was a trip our family will never forget. We still talk weekly about the wish trip. I encourage you to allow your child to make a wish. There are lots of wish-granting programs. If one doesn't grant your child's wish, keep searching. I'm sure you'll find one that will grant your child's specific wish.

Be on your guard against the enemy who seeks to steal, kill and destroy our joy. I warn parents to be aware of feelings of anger or depression on the trip. For me I experienced both. The enemy brings up the past to steal your present joy. I kept thinking about the real reason we were on the trip. Other parents have shared similar thoughts. Some parents who took the trip immediately after diagnosis said that they cried the entire trip, thinking this might be the last fun thing their child would do before he died. This can be one of the most precious memories your child takes into adulthood, enjoy it to the fullest with him. You both are well deserving.

The enemy brings up the past to steal your present joy.

Camp

Camping is as old as humanity. Still today there's something about roughing it that brings out the child in all of us.

As with the wish-granting programs, there are numerous different camping opportunities available. There are camps specific to your child's particular illness, birth defect or injury. There are family camps and sibling camps as well. If one camp doesn't fit your child's needs, keep looking. The variety is endless.

Katie and Ryan attended sibling camp the year after Chad's diagnosis. We left them crying that they didn't want to stay. We dragged them home a week later crying that they didn't want to leave.

This opportunity allowed them to connect with other siblings and to share their feelings about the crisis. Fun and adventure were mixed in to let the kids be kids.

Ryan Brown attends camp annually. In fact, he calls his camp organization each year in January to make sure he gets his application in time. He wouldn't miss it for the world.

32 – Life is a Party

Celebrating the Milestones

> *"Celebrate this as a festival to the Lord for seven days each year." (Leviticus 23:41)*

Celebration is God inspired. He instructed his people, the Israelites, to celebrate as a remembrance of when God brought them out of Egypt. We please God when we thank him in celebration.

Celebration is God inspired. He instructed his people, the Israelites, to celebrate....

Birthdays, Christmas and Easter are days of celebration at our home. Now we have so much more to celebrate. We celebrate the small stuff.

Celebrating began on October 1996, when Dr. K announced that Chad was in remission. Every visit for a bone marrow check demanded a celebration. One month after Buddy, Chad's Hickman catheter, was inserted into his chest, we celebrated Buddy's One Month Birthday. We celebrated when Buddy was taken out of Chad, three years later with a "Going Away Party." This was a miracle. Chad kept one catheter for three years without getting a line infection. I confess that I did go through withdrawals when Buddy left Chad because I fed Buddy heparin 2,190 times.

The big celebration took place on May 19, 1999. Chad's bone marrow was still clear and he went off all treatment. We have annual celebrations every May 19th.

All of this and so much more our family gives thanks to God for and celebrates.

33 – School and Your Child's Individualized Education Plan

Educating the Educators

> *"If any of you lacks wisdom, he should ask God, who gives generously to all without finding fault, and it will be given to him." (James 1:5)*

Some of our greatest battles have taken place in the school conference room during an Individualized Education Plan (IEP) meeting. Working on behalf of our child with the education system may demand a lot of our attention as a parent, but we are our child's best advocates.

It is in our child's best interest if both parents can attend meetings. Two parents united with one mission, to work with the school system in establishing a working education plan for our child with a goal to see our child succeed to the best of his ability, carries weight.

Our first task in working with the principal, teachers and special education area, is that we must educate them about our child and his specific needs. Chad has no physical defects showing he ever had cancer. His healthy appearance serves as a mask to his learning difficulty.

Every school approaches the IEP with its own interpretation of the wording of the IEP as well as how each individual principal and special educator prefers to handle special education.

We experienced a different approach and attitude about the IEP with all six of the elementary schools Chad attended. It's safe to say, I believe I've seen it all. If I haven't seen it all, then I've heard the rest of it from friends who are also dealing with IEPs for their children.

With a working IEP in place, his second grade teacher was content to let Chad fail. She would tell me, "He's failing." In my mind, I thought, *Something is not right here. We have an IEP; he's supposed to be succeeding. What's wrong?* Unreturned phone calls by the principal forced me to do what I knew was best for Chad, pull him out for the second semester to home school him. I began the process before the Christmas break. The day before break Chad got a report card. I told Steve that if he made what I thought he was going to make, I was pulling him out. I opened the envelope to see failing grades in almost every subject. I sent the prepared letter back in with the signed report card on the last day of school before break. That afternoon, I received a phone call from the principal stating that she had received my letter. After informing her that she never bothered to call me back until now, there was nothing to discuss. Chad wouldn't be returning to school.

The home schooling year began in January. Chad was resentful and angry for being pulled out of school. As humiliating as it was for him, he still loved to go to school.

God worked on Chad's behalf. I received a phone call from his special education teacher who also had not bothered to call me before. Since Chad had an IEP in place, we would have to release him from the school or we must continue to bring Chad to school to special education. She said we would need to have another IEP meeting to re-write the IEP.

What a meeting we had. I invited the education consultant, Alma, from the pediatric oncology unit. The room was full. Alma, Steve and I watched in amazement as the princi-

> Chad got a report card. I told Steve that if he made what I thought he was going to make, I was pulling him out.

pal, his 2nd grade teacher who was red-eyed from crying, school psychologist, assistant principal, special education teacher and her supervisor bowed before us for forgiveness and granted any wish we requested.

The truth was that they were in deep trouble and they knew it. The law is on the child's side. This situation should have never happened. I took a drastic step by pulling Chad out to home school him, but talking, or the lack thereof, was getting nowhere. Lesson learned—if you request an IEP meeting, they have to meet. You have the right to invite whomever you deem will be beneficial to your child to provide input. You have the right to request the school system's superiors to the meeting. You have the right to invite the state special education system to the meeting. The teachers and principals do not like to hear these people are attending. The law is on the child's side. Chad completed second grade by being home schooled half the day and attending the special education classroom the other half a day with individualized attention.

Third grade he went back to school. The situation worsened when the students humiliated him. Every time it was time for him to go to special education, the students would say, "Chad, it's time for you to go to special ed." Every day he came home, asking why he had to go to special education and saying that he hated school. Every morning I dropped him off crying and begging me to take him out of special ed. My nerves were frazzled. I completely understood his point of view, but I also knew he needed the extra help. God had a better plan for Chad. He brought about a move to another school through a new job for Steve. We moved from Richmond, Virginia to Abingdon, Maryland.

That was the best thing educationally that ever happened to Chad. I was brainwashed by the previous school to believe that Chad had to be pulled out of the regular classroom to succeed.

At our first meeting with the new principal, I began telling her everything they had done for Chad in the past and what he had to have, or so I wrongly thought.

She listened politely. When I took a breath, she told me that at her school the special educator goes to the classroom and works with all of the students, but particularly paying attention to her students.

His self-esteem skyrocketed. He talked fondly about school. He made honor roll several times. He felt loved and valued. Following fifth grade graduation, I thanked the prin-

> The situation worsened when the students humiliated him. Every time it was time for him to go to special education, the students would say, "Chad, it's time for you to go to special ed."

cipal for believing in Chad. She smiled and answered, "We just saw something in Chad that the other schools didn't see."

Every time we change schools we are forced to tell our story again. God gave me the idea to show the middle school staff where Chad had come from. At our first IEP meeting, I took a tri-fold 3X5 photo holder with the poem, "What Cancer Cannot Do" in the middle, a photo of Chad before diagnosis on one side, and a photo of Chad without hair during treatment on the other side. This visual shows them what Chad fought and survived. Then I tell them Chad's story.

Our goal is to get the educators and principal on our team. Briefly telling the emotional side of our child's story instantly draws more cheerleaders onto his education sideline. Drafting team members who will cheer our child on academically to do his best is our objective as parents.

Chad is 14 years old. He was included at the last IEP meeting. The educators listened to him share how he no longer wishes to be in a classroom with a special educator. I know the day will come when Chad will say, "Enough of special education." I just pray it's after he completes high school.

Sometimes I get weary. I remember what my parents told me, "Enjoy your school years. They are the best years of your life." As Chad's best advocate, it is my goal to see that he enjoys his school years and that they are the best years of his life. He has endured enough unpleasant stuff in life. School will not be an unpleasant area of life for Chad with the Lord's help.

> Drafting team members who will cheer our child on academically to do his best is our objective as parents.

34 – Play

When Can I Start Being a Kid Again?

> *"There is a time for everything and a season for every activity under heaven" (Ecclesiastes 3:1)*

Dr. R told me once, "We all have jobs to do. A preschooler's job is to play. A school age child's job is to go to school."

Chad loved to play in the dirt. A school was being built beside our home. Daily he was in the backyard mimicking the construction equipment with his miniature pieces of equipment.

So long as Ryan cooperated with foreman Chad at the work site everything was rosy. However, one particular afternoon, Ryan apparently had a construction disagreement with Chad. I was just inside the basement loading laundry. I heard a "ka-ting." Next, I heard Chad say, "Oh Bubber, I'm so sorry! Please don't tell Mom!" Not a second later Ryan whaled in pain. Foreman Chad hit Ryan's hand with a child sized metal shovel. It was small, but painful. Chad, in turn, felt pain on his back end.

Chad's working/playing time at the construction site was halted when he had low blood counts. Chad would ask Dr. K after each round of blood work, "Can I dig in the dirt today?" If counts were low, Dr. K would answer, "No Chad, you can't dig in the dirt this week."

However, if counts were good, Chad would ask, "Can I dig in the dirt today?" Dr. K would question, "Do you really have to dig in the dirt, Chad?" Always, his answer was, "Yes, I really need to dig in the dirt." Dr. K would pretend to stab himself in the heart and say, "This is killing me. Okay, Chad, you may dig in the dirt this week." That was a very good week for Chad.

A friend shared an idea of how to bring the dirt pile to Chad in his hospital room. I filled a container with uncooked rice and bought a new miniature construction fleet. Chad moved "dirt" around while lying in the bed. The floor was covered in rice. Chad won the cleaning lady's heart early on in treatment. The first time she came in to clean up the construction zone, I was concerned that she wouldn't be happy. To the contrary, she thought that it was great because it was Chad.

For Christmas he received a 1/16th scale scraper machine. I bought Smarties candy for Chad to scrape up from the bottom of the machine in our entryway. I dug crushed Smarties from the wood crevices with a toothpick for months.

However, he tired of using rice in place of dirt. Nothing filled the longing of his heart but to be outside with real dirt in his hands and all over his clothes. One of his best days was in January. His counts were good and Dr. K gave his blessing on the dirt pile. We bundled Chad up and he spent an hour in his glory. A close up photo reveals a smile on his face and a glow of joy from his heart.

Play is so beneficial to children. It is the informal education setting. Nothing can replace the job of playing for a preschooler. The most memorable of these times was while Chad was playing in the bath water. He was moving water around with construction equipment. I said after allowing him a few minutes play time, "Okay Chad, it's time to get our bath." He looked up at me with sad eyes and asked, "Can't I just play a

> Play is so beneficial to children. It is the informal education setting.

little while longer?" That's when I realized just how much play time he lost over a three-year period. God's truth is that I can't go back and give him those lost years, but I can allow him to play as long as he wants to for the rest of his life.

35 – Survivor's Guilt

The Shadow of Death

> *"Even though I walk through the valley of the shadow of death, I will fear no evil, for you are with me; your rod and your staff, they comfort me." (Psalm 23:4)*

When a friend relapses many parents and children experience survivor's guilt. It is not uncommon to feel guilty that our child is doing well and our friend's child is not. Our prayer is that every child will have a positive outcome and live a long, healthy life. Sadly, statistics tell the truth. Not every child will survive a life threatening illness, birth defect or injury.

We experience survivor's guilt every time a friend's child relapses. Our hearts break for the child and the parents. I talked to Dr. R when one of Chad's friends relapsed. I found myself asking questions such as "Will this happen to my child?" Dr. R stopped me. He said, "Rita, you have to be careful not to attach your cart to his wagon."

This advice goes back to God's truth and the enemy's lie. The truth is that our child is doing well and there's no reason to borrow trouble. The enemy's scheme is to entice us to be fearful that our child will have a setback. He works to steal our present joy by drawing us to dwell on the unknown future. God is not a God of fear. He instructs in the Bible more than anything else, "Do not be afraid." Turn our fears over to God and allow him to quiet this child.

Also, by dwelling on an unknown future, we rob ourselves of time to love our hurting friend and their parents. Although it may be awkward, it is essential to continue being a friend to the child and the parents. We have walked in similar shoes. Remember, we have experienced having friends who do not know what to say and therefore are no longer in touch with us. These parents do not need to feel abandoned by the few friends they do have left.

Again, when contacting these parents following recurrence of disease or the death of their child the most appropriate words are "I am so sorry." Then allow the parents to do the talking while we lovingly listen. Yes, it may be difficult,

> By dwelling on an unknown future, we rob ourselves of time to love our hurting friend and their parents.

Without fail, they always ask me how Chad is doing. It's difficult for me to tell them he is doing well, and I experience survivor's guilt.

but these parents are so appreciative of the friends and family who are there for them during this time. We won't have the answers. We don't need to have the answers. We just need to love them and listen to them.

Each time I make a visit or place a phone call to parents whose child has passed, the parents always thank me. Without fail, they always ask me how Chad is doing. It's difficult for me to tell them he is doing well, and I experience survivor's guilt. However, when I give them the report on Chad, they are always joyful to hear that he is doing well. It's like, although their child lost the battle with this disease, they are glad to hear that someone they know is still fighting and winning the battle.

In caring for our child in this situation, open communication is again crucial. He may be wondering, "Will this happen to me?" This presents an opportunity to share God's truth with our child in a loving way. When one of Chad's friends died at age six, Chad asked me many times to read his obituary out loud. The parents included a sentence saying that the child went to be with the Lord. Chad wanted to know if it meant that he had gone to heaven. I assured Chad many times that the obituary said that he had gone to heaven. Although his friend was gone, this gave Chad hope that someday he would get to see him again and that his friend was completely healed.

36 – Pain Management

Being a Strong Advocate

Advocating for our child in pain is another great role we play. It may be a gentle reminder to the physician asking him to write a prescription for a drug that will counter a certain drug that makes our child extremely sick. It may be as vocal as what one mother did. She could not explain why she had a nagging concern about the number of radiation treatments her son had received for his brain tumor. When the staff followed up on her question, she learned that one more treatment would have caused immediate death. This young man is alive today because his mother listened to the promptings by the Holy Spirit.

No one spends as much time with our child as we do. We have been with them since the beginning of the journey. We've seen how our child reacts to every drug and every pain medicine. We have every right to question a procedure and to ask for another pain medicine when one is not working or has stopped working as well as it once did. We are our child's best advocates.

37 – Thy Will Be Done

The Darkest Valley

No one wants to have experience in this area. This is the area I was most uncomfortable in writing. I prayed, "God, how can I write about parents dealing with their child's death when I haven't experienced this?" He answered, "Rita, I've given you friends who have lost children to disease. They will share their experiences with you." God was so faithful to me. He brought Connie into my life. You met Connie earlier. Her daughter, Michele Diane, passed to her eternal life on May 13, 1996.

During Connie's sharing about the events leading up to Michele's passing, respect for Michele as a person comes through loud and clear. As a mother, Connie chose to allow Michele independence as long as she physically was able to maintain it. During the last hours Connie respected Michele's dignity by asking her, "May I help you?" when Michele was having difficulty doing something on her own.

Connie also continued to celebrate each moment. They held a private high school graduation ceremony for Michele.

Michele's wishes were respected. She did not want to move to a hospice facility. Connie provided full-time care for her. She prayed for wisdom for what practical things to do for her.

Connie also provided spiritual comfort through music and Bible reading. She describes it as "allowing Michele to re-enter her womb—spiritually."

Connie shared that Michele was afraid of pain, not of death. A family friend wrote "Amazing Child, Amazing Creator vs. Amazing Cancellor" about Michele that she read at Michele's memorial service.

Amazing choices! Oh, our amazing child knew in her heart that there was a way for her to conquer this evil one. So she ran straight to him, her Savior! Right into the arms of our amazing creator she flew. And oh, what a whack the old cancellor took. He now had only the power to destroy the outside stuff because the amazing creator had filled our amazing child with a whole new way of living. She totally trusted the amazing creator to provide her every need. And

> He now had only the power to destroy the outside stuff because the amazing creator had filled our amazing child with a whole new way of living.

he did! She ceased being angry, afraid and despairing; now she would not even acknowledge the pain caused by the amazing cancellor's canceling out her physical reserves.

The battle raged. Amazing consequences happened daily. As the cancellor took loveliness of face and figure, the amazing creator gave amazing beauty of soul. The cancellor sapped physical energy—the creator pumped in spiritual energy for prayer and Bible study. The evil one took pleasure in ravaging the body—the creator radiated peace—precious peace. Silently the amazing creator reached out, hugged our amazing child to his loving heart ending the battle for eternity. Rewarding our amazing child with great pride, he provided complete rest, inexpressible joy, unimagined peace and continuous rejoicing. Now she abides with him in love and light, with amazing celebration, forever.

Another important way to respect our child is to allow our child to say goodbye to family and friends the way he wants to. One friend shared how her toddler reached out to every person in the hospital room giving them a hug only minutes before he passed away. She said that she was sure he knew he was going to die and this was his way of saying goodbye.

And when the unthinkable time comes for the child to begin his eternal life—he needs to hear from us that it's okay for him to leave us. This permission says, "It's okay for you to go. God is going to care for you. We'll see you in just a little while." Only God can give us the peace to give our child permission to die and the hope of knowing we will see him again.

Connie says, "At first we pray, 'Thy will be done' idealistically from our head. It's only when we pray, 'Thy will be done' in our heart that the work is complete."

38 – Death—An Outsider's Observations

We Don't Know How We'll React Until We're in that Position

"The Spirit of the Sovereign Lord is on me, because the Lord has anointed me to preach good news to the poor. He has sent me to bind up the brokenhearted, to proclaim freedom for the captives and release from darkness for the prisoners, to proclaim the year of the Lord's favor and the day of vengeance of our God, to comfort all who mourn"
(Isaiah 61:1-2)

If you have experienced the death of your child I want to tell you, "I am so sorry." These four words seem to be among

> Another important way to respect our child is to allow our child to say goodbye to family and friends the way he wants to.

the few that are appropriate when death comes. Other words such as, "I love you" and "I am praying for you" are also appropriate. Although most people are uncomfortable to sit without speaking, just a presence is comforting. Silence allows us to cry and talk, if we want to talk.

If you are at the end of this journey, you may feel relief that the pain is over and that your precious child is no longer suffering. You may feel anger at God that he, in his infinite wisdom, chose not to heal your child on earth. You may just be numb and feel you will never experience life again because of the hole in your life, and the chilling emptiness is more than you want to bear. In a very real sense you have emotionally gone with your child through death. You have answered your child's question, "If I die, will you go with me?" You have walked with him hand in hand to death's door. God has opened the door, in most cases pried your hand from your child's, and then gently and lovingly taken his hand, and closed the door.

Acceptance does not mean that the memory and pain are erased. God made us with emotions and memory. As long as we are in our right mind we will have memory. Also, God has not given us a fast forward button. We remember all. However, only time lessens the memory of pain and heightens the memory of joy you experienced with your child.

The first child I knew who died was a young man in his late teens. James pushed his IV pole up to Chad's door and introduced himself to us. He stopped by during his hallway walks to ask how Chad was doing. He went to Philadelphia for a bone marrow transplant. He did not come home alive. I asked the nurse about him and she shook her head "no" meaning that he did not make it. I glazed down at the floor with tears streaming down my face.

Hearing the death of a child is something we never forget. We met T, a pre-teen, at Dr. K's office. His mother explained that a bone marrow transplant was unsuccessful. Chad went in for a platelet transfusion the night before Father's Day. T was in the room across the hallway. I asked how he was doing. The nurse replied, "Not well." The last words I heard him utter were "Mama help me." I cried.

At 5:30 a.m. his mother awakened me screaming, "NO!" I was paralyzed. She screamed for 15 to 30 minutes. She screamed asking God "Why?" She hit the walls.

Chad's nurse stepped in to check on him. She looked at me. I didn't have to ask but I did anyway, "Did T die?" "Yes,"

If you are at the end of this journey, you may feel relief that the pain is over and that your precious child is no longer suffering.

she said in a quiet, tear-filled cracking voice. My body began to shake as I sobbed uncontrollably. She held me tightly as she comforted me.

I then realized I might think I know how I would respond in that situation but the truth is until we are in that situation we don't have a clue.

Chad was discharged to go home. I couldn't wait to get out of the hospital. I wanted to run out as fast as I could while clutching Chad close to my heart. I placed him beside of me in the bed and said a heartfelt prayer to God, "Thank you, God, for Chad." I kissed his sweet forehead and held him tight. Life is so good. I have everything to be thankful for, and I am.

39 – Keeping the Memories Alive

In Life and Death

> *"And he took bread, gave thanks and broke it, and gave it to them, saying, 'This is my body given for you; do this in remembrance of me.'" (Luke 22:19)*

Jesus instructed a dozen disciples over two thousand years ago to remember him every time they observed Passover. Today, we continue remembering Jesus each time we partake in communion. Keeping memories alive is important to our heavenly Father. One of the greatest gifts from God is that he equipped us with memory. When used the way God intended it, memory is a lifetime blessing. When used the way the enemy intends, it is a haunting nightmare that can cripple us for life.

I enjoy scrapbooking in my spare time. Although sporadic, every time I pull out photos of Chad taken while he was going through his intense treatment phase, I smile. I have been working on Chad's Make-A-Wish® scrapbook since his trip in 2000. It is truly a labor of love.

When I finally returned to work part-time following Chad's diagnosis, my supervisor looked over my shoulder onto my computer background. A friend had scanned Chad's fifth birthday photo and made it my wallpaper on the computer. Although he wore a yellow, plastic hard hat, it was evident that he had no hair. His pale skin told the rest of the story.

My supervisor remarked that one day that would be one of my most treasured photos. He knew from first hand experience since his wife was in remission with non-Hodgkin's

One of the greatest gifts from God is that he equipped us with memory. When used the way God intended it, memory is a lifetime blessing.

Lymphoma. He was absolutely correct. Today it is one of my most cherished photos of Chad. It is a visual reminder of all God has brought Chad and our family through.

Journaling is a wonderful way to preserve memories. Whether written by you or your child, the written word has the ability to transport one back to an event that occurred decades earlier.

There are many other forms of creating memories—drawing, painting or video taping. However, the oldest way of keeping memories alive is through the art of story telling. Since the beginning of time, long before the written language came into being, this was how memories were preserved—through the spoken language.

Each year at Michele's passing anniversary, Connie celebrates Michele's life by taking that day off of work, visiting Michele's grave, reading through Michele's writings, looking at her baby and childhood photos, and talking to friends about Michele's life.

The beauty of Connie's example of how to keep memories alive in death, is that Connie doesn't just remember Michele once or twice a year, but every day. She shares with joy the joy that Michele brought into her life. She keeps Michele's memory alive by sharing Michele with her friends. Although I wasn't privileged to meet her, I feel as though I know her through Connie's fond memories she shares.

I encourage you to keep your child's memories alive by sharing with others your child's story. It will bless others. It will serve as an encouragement to other parents who may just be beginning a similar journey.

I encourage you to keep your child's memories alive by sharing with others your child's story. It will bless others.

Special Needs Ministry

I want to introduce you to three parents of special needs children who have followed God's plan and purpose for their lives.

God grew the Mountain Christian Church Special Needs Ministry through Linda. He prepared her with a Masters in Education and then he gave her the heart for such a ministry through her son, Michael. A nurse friend asked Linda, "When are you going to unwrap the gift that God has given you?" referring to Michael, her special needs child.

While on a family vacation at Sandy Cove, a little boy with autism came to Linda's mind. A voice spoke to her heart, "I die for such as these." She said at that point, "I knew there was going to be a special needs ministry."

It started in 1993. The night before the first special needs ministry Vacation Bible School program, Linda thought about what to say. As she slept, God showed her every turn of her life. The foundation of the special needs ministry was built when Linda was born with a congenital dislocated and deformed left hip. She was in a full body cast for the first two years of life.

Next, she saw a girl digging in the sand on the beach. Her friends asked her to come play, but her response was, "No, I'm searching for treasure."

Linda continued, "That was me. All of my life I was looking for treasure. I was born for this. I always loved the underdog. My gift is treasure hunting. Special needs ministry is treasure that no one else claims. I can look into their eyes and see heaven." Linda is using her gifts, talents, and life experiences for God's kingdom purpose.

Kim was honored as Woman of the Year by the local Civitan club for beginning a sports challenge league for special needs children. Her son, Trey, who was born with Down

Syndrome inspired her to create an avenue for all children to enjoy sports.

Steve Siler has a son with Spina Bifida. He is the founder of Music For The Soul. He says, "I believe the path I have traveled has uniquely prepared me for this endeavor. The mission statement of Music For The Soul is to offer healing, comfort, hope, and encouragement through a series of musical recordings that draw lyrically from the truth of human experience, the inspiration of the scriptures, and the reconciling power of Jesus Christ. I believe firmly and passionately that music is a gift from God and has the power to speak healing straight to people's hearts where words alone can often fail. I truly believe that there are severely hurting people among us who may not be reached any other way but by hearing the message of Christ's renewing love through the gentle touch of music" (www.musicforthesoul.org/default.html).

References

Bagnull, Marlene. *Write His Answer: A Bible Study for Christian Writers*. ACW Press: 1999.

Barg, Gary. *Caregiver.com Newsletter*. Issue 128.

Burkett, Larry. *Hope When It Hurts: A Personal Testimony of How to Deal With the Impact of Cancer*. Moody Publishing: 1998.

Cachiaras, Ben. *The Game of REAL Life: Play it Together Sermon Series*. Mountain Christian Church, January 16, 2005.

Candlelighters Childhood Cancer Foundation. The Quarterly Newsletter. Spring 2002.

CaringBridgeTM. www.caringbridge.org/about.htm

Dockrey, Karen. *When a Hug Won't Fix the Hurt: Walking Your Child Through Crisis*. New Hope Publishers: 2000.

Driscoll, Jean with Janet and Geoff Benge. *Determined to Win: The Overcoming Spirit of Jean Driscoll*. Shaw: 2000.

http://www.jeandriscoll.com.

Focus on the Family. www.family.org.

Leal, Carmen. www.thetwentythirdpsalm.com.

Make-A-Wish Foundation®. www.wish.org.

March of Dimes. www.marchofdimes.com/printable Articles/4439_1026.asp.

Miller, Susan. *NEWComers Connection Newsletter*. Volume 8, Issue 007.

Randall, Tom. *Chapel Message: Grateful People are Happy People*. FCA Golf and Sports Specific Conference, The World Golf Village, St. Augustine, Florida, March 6, 2005.

Samson, Lisa. *Women's Intuition*. WaterBrook Press: October 2002.

Savage, Jill. *Professionalizing Motherhood*. Zondervan: 2001. Used by permission of The Zondervan Corporation.

Scott, Julia. *Coveting the Sky: Finding Your Wings in Depression's Storm*. Atlanta: CarePoint Ministries, Inc., 2005.

Siler, Steve. *Music For The Soul*. www.musicforthesoul.org/default.html.

Stowell, Dr. Joseph. *GriefShare™: Your Journey from Mourning to Joy*. Church Initiative, Inc.: 1999.

Troubledwith.com. www.Troubledwith.com.

World Health Organization. www.who.int/entity/cancer/palliative/en.